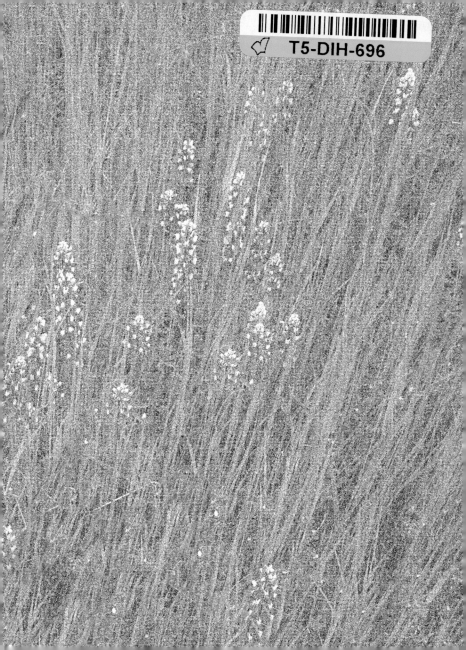

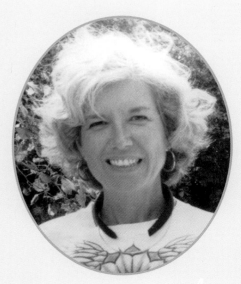

Margaret

Library of Congress
Catalog Card Number 99-66028

ISBN 0-9670683-1-2
Printed in U.S.A.

Bayfield Street Publishing, Inc.

FIRST EDITION

10 9 8 7 6 5 4 3 2 1

Typography and design: Watermark MN Inc.

Editor: Al Chechik

Alan Chechik
RR1, Box 218K
Bayfield, WI 54814
Phone: 715-779-3338
Fax: 715-779-5350
email: artesian@ranger.ncis.net

CREDITS:
Photo of Margaret and Rachael in the dedication: Laura Sunday
Card on page 9: Reprinted with permission of Saga Card Co., Stigler, OK
Card on page 28: Reprinted with permission of Randall Lake, Salt Lake City, UT

REMEMBERING

Margaret

A TRIBUTE

IN THE WORDS

OF SOME

WHOSE LIVES

SHE TOUCHED

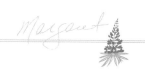

$\mathcal{D}$EDICATION

$\mathcal{M}$om,

Maybe in ten years I'll be able to tell you
what you have meant to my life.
But not quite yet.

I Love You,
Rachael

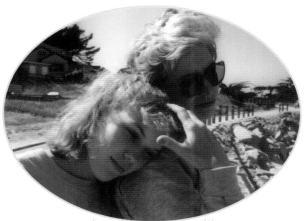

Spring, 1988, Minneapolis

DEDICATION

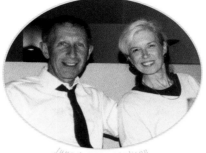

June 4, 1996, Madison

Margaret,
I hope this book will . . .
rekindle warm memories for all who knew and loved you,
introduce you to many who never met you,
help Lucy remember and appreciate the grandmother she knew so briefly,
enable Sonya, Sam– and, perhaps, others later – to learn
about the grandmother they never knew.
Your life defined the book's contents. Your passing inspired its creation.

Forever, Al

Lucy Chechik   *Sonya Chechik*   *Sam Chechik*

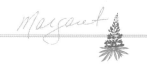

𝒜CKNOWLEDGMENTS

𝒯hank you. . .

TO those who allowed me to use their words in the *Messages* section, and to those who reached into their heart for the *Reflections* section. You have helped the reader understand why Margaret was so special.

TO Roslyn Nelson of Watermark Minnesota Inc. in Minneapolis for designing a book that truly reflects Margaret, and *TO* John Teeter of Bayfield Street Publishing in Washburn, Wisconsin, for helping this book become a reality, and enabling it to happen here in the Chequamegon Bay area. *TO* Shapco Printing, Inc., Minneapolis for a book that I will treasure.

TO you, for acquiring this book. Your purchase tells me that my reasons for preparing it were valid.

TO Regional Hospice in Ashland, Wisconsin and *Sisters of St. Benedict* in Madison, Wisconsin who – each in their own way – offered physical and spiritual assistance during Margaret's illness. They will receive all proceeds from the sale of this book.

Alan Chechik
Bayfield, Wisconsin, Summer, 1999

REFACE

June 30, 1998, 1:20 p.m.

As I begin to put thoughts on paper that I know will change
many times before they're finalized, I'm following a routine
I acquired in junior high – lying on my bed, writing in longhand.
I know it's bad for the back, and I'm sure educators frown on it.
But it works for me.

During high school and college days in Madison, I had only my
bedroom walls to gaze at while writing or doing homework. Today,
I'm looking out my bedroom window over a sea of trees lush with
summer vegetation toward a small, blue sliver of Lake Superior.

I'm in the loft of my home in Bayfield, Wisconsin.
I've been its only resident for nearly three years.
I had shared it with my wife, Margaret.

We planned the loft – about 500 square feet – as our private retreat
in a home we hoped would often be filled with guests: a bed and
breakfast. The loft, under an A-frame roof, has a bed, a sitting area,
two closets, an office area, and a bathroom.

And light, lots of light: four windows looking north and less than
10 feet from being in the woods; six skylights – three each facing
east and west; two large windows and french doors looking south.
Our bed faced the eastern sky. At night we would lie and watch the

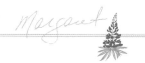

stars slowly appear and grow bright. Then, as dawn approached –
and we often found ourselves awake at the same time – the stars
dimmed, slowly faded, disappeared. Sometimes we were silent;
sometimes we voiced our innermost thoughts about the
fading of the stars and what was happening in our lives
in the late summer of 1996.

As I look toward the lake, I'm asking myself: Why would anyone
want to own a book composed of sympathy notes and personal
recollections related to the death of someone they had never met?
Had never even heard of?

Why? Because four months ago I re-read – for the first time
in 15 months – the contents of a large box filled with such
messages and realized I was looking through a small treasure . . .
notes that capture the intensely personal feelings and emotions that
linger inside all of us in connection with special people
in our life . . . feelings and emotions that we may not discover
and be able to express unless – and, sadly, until – that special
person is taken from us.

Every card shop is testimony that most of us struggle for words
when we try to express deep feelings in writing. So we rely
on Hallmark and American Greetings to choose those words
for us. And we sign our name and mail it. And feel a little
better. And perhaps the recipients gain some small
comfort from these notes.

My loss was Margaret.

The treasure I found was in re-reading personal words that complemented – yes, transcended – the cards' printed messages. Words written by close friends and colleagues, by people who had known her for many years, just briefly, or in some cases, had never met her.

I tell myself this is something that needs to be done. As a tribute to Margaret . . . as a thank you to those who shared their feelings . . . to give life to the beauty of the sentiments people are able to express over a loss . . . perhaps to help others facing the loss of a loved one . . . as a powerful reminder to say the things that need to be said while those special people in our lives are with us . . . and, certainly, as a measure of healing for myself.

So. . . some background . . .

Margaret and I were married June 16, 1985 in Madison, Wisconsin. I was 50; she was 38. I had two sons, Marc, 24, and Joel, 21, by a previous marriage. She had a daughter, Rachael, 11, by a previous marriage. Some would call it an unlikely match. She was born and raised in a Catholic home in Little Chute, WI, a town of about 9,000 halfway between Appleton and Green Bay. I was born and raised in a Jewish home in Madison, the state capital. Unlikely, but it worked.

Margaret was employed in public relations for Kenosha (WI) Memorial Hospital at the time we were married. I worked in the same field for the Wisconsin Hospital Association

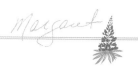

in Madison. She continued to live and work in Kenosha
until late summer to complete her job. Rachael and I lived
together in our condominium in Madison. When Margaret joined
us permanently, she had accepted a position as Marketing Director
for Smith and Gesteland, a large Madison CPA firm.
The job was newly-created, in part by a new focus
on marketing in the accounting field,
and in part by the fit with Margaret's communication and personal
skills – products of her experience in health care public relations
and her Executive MBA acquired through the University
of Wisconsin-Milwaukee's two-year, weekend program while
a single parent, working at Kenosha Memorial.

Over the next 11 years, she would use her skills in a variety
of professional, community and personal relationships, activities
and projects. In the early 1990s she would leave the CPA firm,
form her own marketing consulting firm, join the faculty of
Milwaukee-based Cardinal Stritch College and work with
the Small Business Development Center at the
University of Wisconsin in Madison.

Because of the 12-year difference in our ages, we talked often
about my taking early retirement in the mid-1990s. By the late
1980s, we had begun to discuss the idea of opening a bed and
breakfast, which seemed to offer an attractive opportunity
to meet interesting people and create our own special lifestyle
while generating adequate income to support us.

We spent many summer weekends during 1991 and 1992 exploring towns in northern Wisconsin that might fulfill Margaret's criteria for a successful B&B location: a tourist destination, on big water, with reliable snow. The search narrowed to the farthest reaches of northwest Wisconsin – Bayfield, a town of less than 700 on the south shore of Lake Superior.

We originally planned to buy an existing B&B or an older home that could be converted to a B&B. But the combination of older homes and Margaret's asthma made this impossible.

The alternative was to buy land and build. We bought 24 acres just south of Bayfield in the summer of 1994, dug the driveway that fall, designed the house that winter with the help of a husband-wife designer team near Madison, contracted with a Bayfield builder and broke ground June 15, 1995.

Margaret moved into the nearly-completed house in April, 1996 to keep watch on final construction. I remained in Madison to complete my job. We sold our condo in May, and I moved in with a dear (female) friend of Margaret's in Madison. Rachael, then 22, had graduated from college and was off on her own, also in Madison. Margaret came to Madison June 4 for my retirement party. I retired on Wednesday, June 12, packed and drove to Bayfield on June 13, and, along with Margaret, welcomed our first guests June 14, 1996.

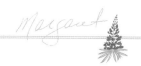

Our nearly six years of careful planning had been successful.
The Artesian House, the bed and breakfast we
nurtured from an obscure vision – a sketch on a piece
of graph paper – had become reality.

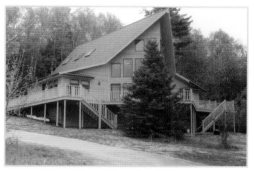

Our new home, June, 1996

Less than six weeks later, Margaret was diagnosed with inoperable
stomach cancer. She died October 20, 1996 at age 49.

At our wedding in 1985, we exchanged watches instead of rings.
As we explained to the small gathering of friends and family
during the ceremony: "The only thing you have together is time."

And time, as we learned, can be a fickle friend.

The thoughts expressed in this book were taken from among
hundreds of cards received following Margaret's death.
They reveal the depth of the sentiments that friends and
acquaintances found in their hearts.

When I decided to prepare this book, I wrote to each person whose words I wanted to borrow, told them my plans and asked permission to use their message. Not one declined. I also wrote to a small group – family, Margaret's close friends and colleagues, plus a few who became intimate acquaintances as a result of her illness. I invited them to write a memory or a recollection.

The result is *"Remembering Margaret."*

I was privileged to be part of her life for one-third of her 49 years. That she was unique in many ways, to many people, is apparent from the words you will read. Virtually everything that could be said about her qualities is stated one way or another in this book

...Except for this:

When people are taken in their prime – without warning – we ask "why?" When I posed this to one of Margaret's closest friends – Karen Julesberg, whose reflection you will read – she smiled and said, "Her work was done."

I am learning to accept that.

Alan Chechik, Bayfield, Wisconsin, July 20, 1999

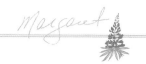

$\mathscr{O}$NTRODUCTION TO MESSAGES

This section contains some of the messages received after Margaret's death on October 20, 1996. In a few cases the message was sent just prior to her passing, and that is noted. These messages came from family, friends, professional colleagues, guests at The Artesian House and a few who had only met Margaret briefly, or had never met her.

I requested permission from each person whose words I wanted to borrow. All said "yes." Each person was given the option to be identified by full name, first name and initial, or first name only.

These messages are reproduced as originally written. In some cases, I have omitted the names of people, companies or other information that I felt may have detracted a bit from the message itself. A few have been shortened slightly for space. Where appropriate, I have included a few explanatory words to clarify. They appear in parentheses and in italics. And, wherever possible, I have added a few words (in italics) to help you understand the writer's relationship with Margaret.

Al Chechik

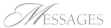

MESSAGES

We were stunned to hear the news of Margaret's passing.
She had so much life and vitality! Her spirit and love will
definitely live on in every corner of The Artesian House and
in the lives of the guests. Mom and I feel honored to have shared
your opening week excitement. She enjoyed the book, *Fireweed*,
that Margaret recommended, and we often eat yogurt with granola
on top! Her caring for others was real – remember her driving
a couple of hours to pick up the piano player whose car broke
down? Your love for each other was so evident and real.
Thank you for your example of a life lived fully and in the present.

Joan Sundberg, St. Paul, MN
a guest, with her mother, the second weekend the B&B was open

Margaret was so vibrant and alive. I have an image of her
leading lively, heavenly discussions, making new friends and
planting new gardens. Her spirit will live on – I'm sure of it.

(What follows is from a card sent by the Heils two weeks before Margaret's death)
You are in our prayers constantly. We hope you are having
more good days than bad and that all the really
important thoughts are being spoken.

Donna and Marty Heil, Verona, WI – our first guests, June 14, 1996
Donna is an avid gardener.

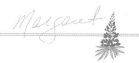

*W*e received your letter yesterday, and there is no way
to express how sad we were to learn that Margaret had passed
away. Even though we knew you as guests of your wonderful
B&B for such a short time, we both looked upon you as friends.
We stayed with you for the second time the weekend of July 20th,
which would have been just a few days before Margaret
was diagnosed. I wasn't aware that she was having health
problems – she certainly did not appear to be ill.
It was such a shock to read your letter.

It is so ironic that during the past several weeks I thought
of you often, wondering how your first season was and what
you would do over the winter. We actually tried to plan another
trip the weekend after Apple Fest, but with our work and travel
schedules we were not able to pull it off.

So many times we have talked to our friends about the
wonderful B&B we found in Bayfield. We have many warm
memories of our visits with you. . .eating ice cream at 10 p.m.
with you and Margaret in your kitchen and those two-hour-long
breakfasts with you and the other guests.

We want you to know that our thoughts are with you.

Louise and Alex Palmer, Minnetonka, MN – guests in June, 1996
who returned for a second stay a month later

$\mathscr{I}$ was so very sorry to receive your news about Margaret.
I had just begun thinking about her comment this summer about
adding us to your Christmas card list. I was anticipating getting
our first one from you and sending one in return.
You certainly will be on our list this year. I'll miss Margaret's news.

She was such a special lady, and we very much enjoyed
our three days with you both this summer. I'm glad you plan
to keep The Artesian House going.

Sally, Normal, IL – B&B guest with her husband, Todd, July, 1996

$\mathscr{S}$ ally and I have often talked and reflected on our wonderful
time in Bayfield this past summer. And you and Margaret were
definitely the highlight of our trip. We feel very blessed that we
had the opportunity to spend some time with you. Now we truly
understand how timely our visit and stay with you was.
Sally and I hope to return to The Artesian House some day, and
I'm certain Margaret's spirit and sense of humor will be present.

Todd, Normal, IL

$\mathscr{I}$ want to express my deepest sympathy to the ending
of Margaret's "life's journey," as expressed in the moving obituary.
I was the OB nurse who talked to her in the hospital, and got her
in touch with *(local hospice director)*. I was deeply moved by the
brief times she and I spent together and by her very loving family.

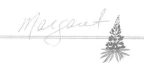

I wanted to let you know that when I read in the paper that
she had passed away, I had a clear sense that her spirit
was with me, waiting for me to find that out; and she gave
me a hug and thanked me and left.
Somehow I feel that her spirit is continuing its journey even now,
and if it's possible to be on the "other side" and yet be with the
ones you loved on Earth, then a part of Margaret is still with you.

*Jan Perkins, R.N., Ashland, WI – A nurse at Memorial Medical Center
who connected briefly, but powerfully, with Margaret*

(dated one week before Margaret's death)
*D*ear Margaret,

I'm sorry we all don't have more time with you.
This horrible cancer is whisking you away too quickly.
It hurts me to think that I won't be able to see you, but I know
you need to save your strength for your family.
I'm angry that God has allowed someone as strong and dynamic
to be taken over by cancer. I'm disappointed that we haven't had
time together, with long, quiet walks and time for reflection.
But, I'm grateful that we found each other in Madison nearly
10 years ago, and that we've shared a beautiful, caring friendship.
There is no one on earth that knows me as well as you do.
You have a gift for probing into the hearts and minds of others,
learning about them, yet not being judgmental. You have been my
mentor, my friend, my confidante and I shall miss you dearly...

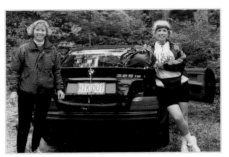

Julie Pedretti, left, and Margaret on one of their many adventures.

...Yesterday was a day to enjoy nature. It was the kind of day we both love, and several years ago we would have found a long trail for a hike. I spent part of the day washing the cars, carrying firewood and sweeping the leaves off the patio – I thought of you all day and cried. It's so selfish...It's so difficult to accept that we won't be enjoying those days together again.

Julie Pedretti, Milwaukee, WI – She and Margaret were professional colleagues and close friends who shared a love for hiking, biking, sailing, camping and cross-country skiing

*W*e all lost a great spirit in Margaret. It was as if she was plucked out of thin air. She enabled me to come to my physical home, Madison, and my spiritual home, St. Benedict Center. I'm so very thankful to her. We'll miss her jaunty stride, her beatific smile and her witty style.

Marykay Bell, a friend and professional colleague, who Margaret helped attract to a position at St. Benedict Center in Madison, WI

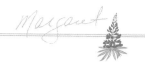

$\mathcal{W}$e were so sorry to hear from you about Margaret's death.
My daughter and I thought she was a lovely and elegant woman.
I remember her vibrant and sparkling eyes, and now that
I know what she was going through at the time we were there –
I know how, indeed, courageous she was.

Carole Gealow, Mankato, MN – a guest in August, 1996 with her daughter, Kendra

$\mathcal{I}$ was so sorry to hear the news from my mother about your
wife's death. I first saw what an elegant woman she was when
I saw the pictures of her in your photo album. Of course her
elegance was more vivid in person. She was the special kind
of person that one always remembers meeting.

I admire you both for having fulfilled a dream together of
opening a bed and breakfast. Not many people can say they
have succeeded in following their dreams in life.

You are very fortunate in this way. Even though it may have been
unfairly cut short, you had a beautiful place to enjoy together.
Know that someone touched by your kindness and hospitality
last summer is now thinking of you from across the ocean
(the Netherlands) and wishing you the very best.

Kendra Gealow

$\mathcal{I}$t's funny, but for some reason my heart this evening (*Margaret's memorial service in Madison 11/2/96*) was filled with joy and a wonderfully calm feeling about Margaret. I'm not usually this peaceful about these matters. But I've been able to look back and remember Margaret with such respect and delight. What a force of energy! I've also had the chance to chuckle over our younger years of dancing and sitting in the whirlpool. Not stuff that's proper to mention at a memorial service. But it's all there – forever captured in our hearts and memories.

JoAnne Sturiale, Madison, WI – a friend and professional colleague, who, with Margaret, enjoyed the "social side" of meetings of Wisconsin hospital public relations people

$\mathcal{N}$eedless to say, Creighton and I were shocked to hear the news about Margaret! I, too, have had breast cancer, and my husband died of brain cancer earlier this year, so I know how devastating these experiences can be. I'll always remember the great time we had at your B&B; it was a happier time. Margaret was a sweet soul and we will remember her with fondness. Creighton and I will be married on June 14, 1997 in a big ceremony overlooking our lake. We are very excited to formally begin our new life!

Creighton and Linda Cox, Embarrass, MN – guests one week after we opened, who announced their engagement at breakfast just before they left for home.

As the weekend service approaches *(to commemorate the first anniversary of Margaret's death and dedicate her marker in Madison on October 20, 1997)*, we want to send our love and thoughts. As I said earlier in October, regardless of where family is next Saturday, we're all with you in spirit and sharing our hopes for renewal as you honor our Margaret. The picture on this card from Santa Fe reminded me of Margaret – she is leaving her

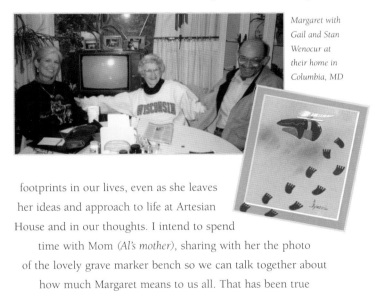

Margaret with Gail and Stan Wenocur at their home in Columbia, MD

footprints in our lives, even as she leaves her ideas and approach to life at Artesian House and in our thoughts. I intend to spend time with Mom *(Al's mother)*, sharing with her the photo of the lovely grave marker bench so we can talk together about how much Margaret means to us all. That has been true many times – and will always be true.

Gail (Al's sister) and Stan Wenocur, Columbia, MD – Gail and Stan cut short a west coast vacation to run the B&B during Margaret's initial chemotherapy in August, 1996.

My sister and I stayed with you this past summer, the weekend that Margaret was in Madison. I had the pleasure of meeting her earlier in the summer when we toured Artesian House. I am very saddened to hear of Margaret's death, so sudden and unexpected. I know that Artesian House is the result of a shared vision.

Catherine Koemptgen, Duluth, MN – a published photographer/author and guest in July, '96

We never had the privilege of meeting Margaret, but just hearing you speak of her and seeing her obvious influence on the serenity and charm of The Artesian House, we know she must have been a very special lady. You touched our hearts by your kindness and hospitality when you surely had other things on your mind. It is said that although scars remain, the wounds will heal. May the Lord surround you with comfort, love and peace.

Paul and Deb Mahacek, Eden Prairie, MN – the last guests, Oct. 6-7, 1996
before we closed to devote our time totally to Margaret's care.

All of us at Smith & Gesteland have been troubled and saddened by Margaret's loss. She made significant contributions to the people and projects which she touched. It is extremely difficult to understand why she has been taken at a time and stage in life when dreams are just being realized. I wanted to write and say thank you to you and Rachael for sharing her with us and our firm. I learned a great deal from her, and my life has been

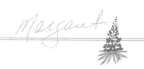

enriched by knowing her as a colleague and a friend. Her love
of life, enthusiasm and advocacy of others are among the
memories I shall have of her. Hopefully, your memories will bring
you some comfort at this time. Margaret was loved by many,
and she served as a willing mentor and inspiration for several
of us. For that, I am truly grateful. It is my hope that the Lord
has found a special place for her spirit.

*Scott Braucht, Madison, WI – a colleague at the CPA firm who worked
closely with Margaret on many projects*

Written to Al and Rachael

$\mathscr{A}$ is with such sadness, shock and disbelief that I write this
card to you. I have never met either of you, but I have heard about
you both over the years from Margaret, who I met a number
of years ago when we hired her to do consulting for the company
I worked for. I was immediately drawn to her charm, wit, sparkle,
warmth, intelligence, genuineness, and so many other things...
...Over the years we kept in touch, had lunch several times,
and we hired her again when she had her own consulting
business. She was one of the finest people I have ever met, and
I will always cherish the time that I was able to spend with her.
I am so honored she touched my life.
Margaret was the rarest of gifts to us all!!

Candi, Madison, WI – a professional colleague who became a friend

$\mathscr{I}$don't have words for how I know Margaret ... my memory
is of feelings and a very special sense of aliveness and love,
Margaret-style ... rolled up in it is our last week together,
a closing chapter of the Margaret of Gesundheit days ...
it's a joy to know Margaret within me.

*John Rubel, Renick, WV – He and Margaret became close friends during our
trip to West Virginia in 1990, and the friendship was renewed during subsequent
visits in 1991 and 1992. John spent a week with us in Bayfield a month before Margaret's death.*

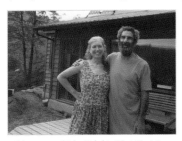

Margaret and John Rubel in West Virginia.

$\mathscr{T}$o say I was taken a bit by surprise would certainly
be an understatement. Somehow we always seem to think
we have time to renew and nurture long-term friendships.

Margaret was a special human being. Somehow we always bridged
the gaps that seemed to dominate our friendship.
Always too much distance, not enough time.

Margaret

I met her at a lunch in January, 1984. She was stressed because
of all that was going on at the hospital. She and a few others were
handling the union campaign about 24 hours a day. Despite
it all, she was energized, vibrant, bright and oh so humorous.
What a wonderful cynical wit!! From that point on, she and
I always had fun ribbing one another. She could take it and dish
it out. I was privileged to know her. A wonderful woman. I always
admired her strength, independence, heart, her love of Rachael
and how important you were in re-shaping her life
as she considered leaving Kenosha.

Her dream was to open a B&B in northern Wisconsin.
I'm so very happy she was able to do it.

_Russ Jones, Winfield, IL – a consultant who first met Margaret while she was in
Kenosha. They stayed in touch periodically after she moved to Madison._

You and your family have been in my thoughts since Margaret's
memorial service on Saturday. I didn't know Margaret very well,
but the woman remembered in that service was the one I knew –
and I suspect the same was true for all her friends there. I always
thought of that as Margaret's greatest gift – you knew her, knew
who she was, right away – and she presented such enthusiasm
and no apologies. It was my honor to know her briefly.

_Ellen Kennedy, Madison, WI – She and Margaret became acquainted
while Margaret was working with the sisters at St. Benedict Center._

$\mathcal{M}y$ thoughts have been with you since I heard the horrible
news of Margaret's illness and death – still difficult
to comprehend. My last recollection was at your retirement party
(June 4, 1996), and shortly before when I ran into Margaret
at a Madison shop. She was full of excitement and enthusiasm for
the new venture you both were about to begin – sharing photos
and stories of The Artesian House in progress. I also have a vivid
memory of your brief tribute to Margaret at your retirement party
– the love, pride and respect were so evident. I hope you can find
comfort in the beauty of Bayfield, support of many caring friends
and family and treasured thoughts and memories.

Priscilla Arsove, Madison, WI – a friend and professional colleague
from Margaret's days in hospital public relations

$\mathcal{L}$eo and I were overcome with sadness when we read your lovely
ad in the County Journal and realized that Margaret had died.
We briefly met the two of you last summer when you graciously
showed us Greg Carrier's handiwork. *(He built The Artesian House.)*
Somehow, we felt bonded to you immediately – maybe this
happens with all your visitors and B&B guests –
and when we saw your Shalom Menorah in the kitchen,
we wondered if you might be the only two others in Bayfield
who would know how to light the candles with us. I would have
loved to have known Margaret – her warmth and generosity were

evident from the moment we met. Perhaps we will come to know
her in spirit, through you. Greg must be glad, now, that he
moved that skylight, for it surely gave her great pleasure
to take in the view from her bath.

Chris and Leo Stern, Minneapolis, MN
They met Margaret just once – while touring our B&B.
They built a home in Bayfield with Greg Carrier as general contractor.

*T*his is a note I've been trying for weeks to write . . .
I wanted to find words better than the ones in my mind
to tell you how sad and sorry the news of your wife's death made
me. Many times over the past year I thought of you two with more
than a touch of envy – that lovely little inn you created –
the fun of taking an idea, a dream, and making it real.
A quieter time in a quieter town.
It was clear to me how much of yourselves you poured into it all.
I don't know where you land on the subject of faith . . . mine is
always shaken when people go through what you have . . . the why
of it. There is no why. I know you'll come through this,
and I have to believe there's another plane of happiness that you'll
reach. If it isn't to be found for someone like you,
well then my faith is truly shaken.

Rick Wade, Arnold, MD
a professional colleague and friend of Al's for more than 15 years, who never met Margaret

𝒟ear Margaret,

𝒲e were shocked and saddened to learn of your illness. The world is certainly not fair when someone as kind and full of life as you are must suffer. John and I wanted to let you know that we always looked forward to your classes when we were in school. You were by far the most informative, upbeat and entertaining instructor we had at Cardinal Stritch. You also helped us tremendously with our (*equivalent of a final thesis.*) We couldn't have done it without you. It is because of your expert advice about our papers that we are now official MBA graduates. It was never easy with both of us working and trying to raise a baby. Speaking of babies, our new daughter is doing just fine. Margaret is now 4 1/2

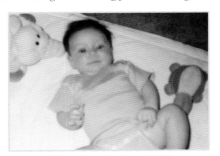

Margaret Ryan, born June 7, 1996

months old and is starting to move on her own a little bit. Her big brother, Adam, is a bit jealous of her, but he is adjusting. We chose the name Margaret for our baby because we know two Margarets who are inspiring to us and whom we admire

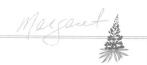

very much. You, of course, are one of them, and the other
is a friend of John's family who raised eleven kids, all of whom
are successful in their own way. She is the most successful mother
we know, and you are the most successful career woman we know.
Our little Margaret is sure to be successful in whatever she chooses
to do with her life. Margaret, we had to let you know that you made
a difference in our lives and we feel lucky to have shared time
with you. Our thoughts and prayers are with you.

John and Tamara Ryan, New Lisbon, WI – students in the MBA class
Margaret taught for Cardinal Stritch College

August 17, 1996

*D*ear Margaret,

We have only met briefly about 6 months ago, but I feel
as if I know you. *(Mutual friend)* has kept me up to date on your
health and has shared what has happened to you. I, of course, can
understand a little more deeply what you are going through because
of my own health situation. I think the first time I saw you I was
knee deep into my chemotherapy and wearing hats and scarves.
I don't know too well what your present situation is with treatment
etc., but I just wanted to let you know that I think of you often.
There is something about having cancer that binds those who are
dealing with it firsthand and brings others closer. I have experienced
much love and compassion from so many people throughout this
year; *(mutual friend)* has been especially wonderful to me. I can only...

...imagine that she has the same love and compassion for you.

And I am so sorry that you are going through this! In between chemotherapy and radiation treatments, I went to Mexico. On the last day of my trip, I met a woman who had had a brain tumor and was told she had a 1% chance of surviving. Against all odds, she went through surgery to have it removed and is still alive one year later. We exchanged addresses and have been corresponding ever since. I relate this story because of the uniqueness of the relationship. I can talk to the woman like I can with no other person. For some reason, I can open up and let her know about fears and sadness that no one else can hear. Maybe it's because I really don't know her. Maybe it's because she lives in Texas. Maybe I can open up more when I write as opposed to speaking directly; it's safer. If you want to correspond, I would like that. If not, I completely understand and only want what is best for you. If nothing more, at least you know that I am thinking of you and wish you the best. I hope you come to terms with your illness and find peace, whatever your circumstance.

Michelle Moan, Madison, WI
Michelle wrote this letter based on one brief meeting with Margaret.

$\mathscr{I}$ extend my deepest sympathy at your loss of Margaret. I met her only a few times but sensed such excitement, energy and charm. She must have been a wonderful life partner. For the Chautauqua Board, I thank you for listing the *Big Top* as a recipient of memorials. We had hoped to involve Margaret and you in our activities as you became more settled here. We hope you will stay and that we will see

more of you next summer. Reading that beautiful obituary again
I feel this community suffers a loss when so talented and delightful
a lady was whisked away before we could truly enjoy her.
Again, please accept the sympathy of a Bayfield neighbor.

Kitty Hartnett, Bayfield, WI – local resident, active in the arts, who had met Margaret just briefly

We met when I dropped off cider the morning of your open house.
My daughter and I were enchanted with your wife and with her creative
enjoyment of your place in Bayfield. Her many references to cross country
skiing plans make the sudden death even more poignant.
I never fail to think of you as I pass your place on my way home
from work. Your loss is also the community's loss.

Dawn and Einar Olsen, Bayfield, WI – local orchard operators who met Margaret once or twice

I've re-read the obituary of Margaret's several times and will probably
keep it a long time. I never met her, but I can see her spirit through the
words written in that column. The things that were significant to her are
important to me, too. I'm sorry I missed knowing her. I'm sure she made
a real, beneficial impact on anyone she came in touch with.
Her time in the Bayfield area was too short, I think. I know you'll see
these things that spoke to her all around you up here.
I certainly will. She is a great reminder to relish life.

*Kathleen Russell, Bayfield, WI – a local realtor with special interest
in outdoor and environmental activities*

The writer of this letter survived colon cancer in 1989.
She never met Margaret, but has a strong spiritual sense and handed this letter
to Al at a small memorial service held for Bayfield area friends
on November 30, 1996.

*M*y beloved husband, lover and friend, I am in a place of
newness that is quite something! It cannot be described in earthly
terms, but it's all I had hoped for. Many welcome us here including
some that you and I have known. It is difficult to see you sad.
I know you are trying hard. Be stilled by the knowledge that I live
in spirit. This may not help now, but as time unfolds, you will know
deeply in your heart that it is so. You may believe that we are apart,
but the paradox is that I have never been so close! I will not be
in a physical place, yet all things are connected in astounding ways.
The truth of our love is the truth of all love. Isn't that sublime?
I will not be able to speak with you directly for a while, but that
may come too. So know, my dearest man, how fortunate we have
been. We lived so much in those eleven blessed years. Let your life
now be dedicated to raising your own consciousness and serving
all you meet. I have loved you so. It is forever, you know. Be glad
and celebrate who we have been. I will take my leave now.

Trust this new friend who brings this to you. She understands
the truth of who we all are. I am always – your love – Margaret
P.S. I almost forgot. Don't forget to tend the plants.

Diane Brander, Washburn, WI and Sheridan, MT

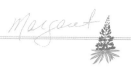

This e-mail message was received October 16, 1996,
four days before Margaret's death.

$\mathscr{D}$ear Margaret and Al,

E-mail seems a bit impersonal, but I don't want to interfere
with the time you have together right now. Margaret, my mom,
passed on your final good-bye, and I want to pass on my
own good-bye to you. We didn't have much time
together, but what we did have I enjoyed deeply (I
remember sailing in Madison on your little boat. I think
I've finally learned port from starboard; or was that bow
from stern?) I feel like we've created a strong connection
in a short time. I find it hard to make sense of the
unfairness of your illness and impending death. Studying
Tai Chi and Chi Gung and Taoist ideas has helped me to believe
in the necessary relationship of life and death, that these are
two sides of the same thing. I find this comforting – death,
even a cruel and unfair one
– is part of life. Something else which Taoists strongly believe is that
the best way to help a person with their death, and to help yourself,
is to resolve your connection to that person so they are free to die,
so that their life is completed. This doesn't mean forgetting that
person, or not missing them, but letting them go.
So, from whatever our connection is, I let you go. Good bye.

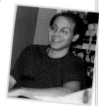

Jonathan Wenocour

Jonathan Wenocur, Belmont, MA
Al's nephew and Margaret saw each other only a few times
but developed a strong attachment.

$\mathcal{I}$ am so sorry to hear about Margaret's passing.
She impressed me from the moment I met her. I'm sure you
know the feeling. She taught me – showed me is a better way
to put it – what mentoring means – more than a buzzword.
I wish I could have been more a part of these last months,
learning the hardest lessons.

*Sarah White, Madison, WI – a professional colleague and friend of Margaret's
who designed The Artesian House logo.*

$\mathcal{I}$ 've written this letter over and over in my head, but couldn't
bring myself to put it on paper. As I "wrote" it – I kept
remembering my time with Margaret. I can't believe my luck
when she helped me put together our first programs in Family
Business while at Smith & Gesteland. Then there was our bagel
breakfast. That was when she told me she was going to put her
life in balance and go out on her own. I know the best thing
I've done in my tenure was to say "let us be one of your clients,
come work with us – you name the conditions." She became our
biggest asset. She worked with many small businesses and always
made a difference. But she made a difference to the *core* of the
organization. She helped with our search and screens, supported
(colleague) and me with her sage advice and saw me through the

worst year of my life. When she moved up north, she left a huge void but I knew she was only a call away. I keep going back to the words I've repeated all my life, that our loved ones "live on in the acts of goodness they perform and in the hearts of those who cherish their memories." With all the wonderful acts of goodness Margaret performed, she'll be remembered, and as long as we draw breath, she will be with us.

Joan Gillman, Madison, WI – a colleague and friend
who shared professional highs and lows with Margaret

*H*er dancing eyes and embracing smile seemed to radiate Margaret's love for the natural world. She was a gift to us all.

Libby Telford, neighbor and first friend in Bayfield, WI

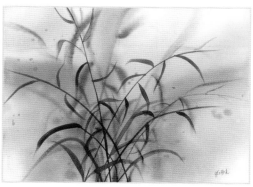

Libby's husband, John, an avid gardener and painter, immediately connected with Margaret through their shared love of flowers. John painted this watercolor for her and delivered it — with tears in his eyes. He inscribed it: "To Margaret, for her love of grasses and her indomitable spirit."

I feel a deep sense of loss and sadness at Margaret's death.
At the same time, I am grateful that she now rests in God's love.
All her pain is past. I served on the committee that recommended
her as a consultant to the Sisters of St. Benedict. She was a model
for many of us. I will always remember her incredible insights
and curiosity about life and people. But most of all,
I will remember how her face lighted up when she mentioned
your name and the things you did together.
You were the apple of her eye.

Kathleen K, a colleague who knew Margaret through St. Benedict's, Madison, WI

*O*f course, I was stunned to hear of Margaret's transition.
I loved her bravado, gutsiness, humor and sharp/quick responses.
She'd say things that no one else had the courage to say.
(There's a bit of that in me, too). When my Mom committed
suicide in '93, many wouldn't talk to me directly. Margaret
did and knew what to say. You are a special spirit to have shared
Margaret's life. I send you healing and love.
Whenever you hurt, remember it's showing you
how deeply you love her.

*Ann P, Chicago, IL – a friend and colleague
through the Chicago-based American Marketing Assn.*

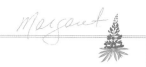

$\mathcal{D}$ear Margaret,

I'm sitting here thinking of you and just wanted to tell you –
which I maybe never did – what a wonderful influence you have
been and still are in my life. You taught me so darn much and
also helped me gain that much-needed confidence in myself.
Also, if it weren't for you and your boating with *(mutual friend)*,
I'd probably not have the great job and boss I do now. Also,
thinking back, one of my favorite things I learned while working
for you was that flowers still come in boxes. You know, the big
long boxes with the big bows. You're the only person I know
who sends flowers in boxes – really classy!
I've got a few prayers going on down at this end.

Marilyn Pertzborn, Middleton, WI – Margaret's secretary at Smith & Gesteland,
who later accepted another position in Madison with some "urging" from Margaret

Written to Margaret prior to her death

$\mathcal{J}$ust a short note to let you know that you are in our thoughts
and prayers. It was nice talking with you and Al last week.
The two of you sounded upbeat, and I'm confident that positive
attitude will bode well for both of you as you battle
your formidable foe.
As a firm believer in the "law of karma," I have no doubt
that you will prevail in this fight to regain your health.
You've done a lot of good for a lot of other people. That...

...unselfish approach to life, coupled with your strong determination, sounds like a recipe for recovery. The morning before I found out about your illness, I was thinking about you and how you served as the catalyst for what is now a very successful fundraising operation. Not only that, but thanks to your guidance, I've been able to work with other neighborhood centers to develop

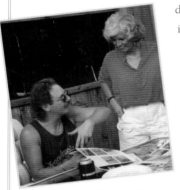

direct mailings which have helped bring in substantial funds for youth programs at other centers. I recall that you came to the Center's rescue in January, 1987 when we were facing a financial crisis. Your leadership and skill in developing a strategic plan to "save" the Center was successful and has truly proven to be "the gift that keeps on giving."

When she moved to Madison in 1985, Margaret renewed an early '70s friendship with Tom Moen. The friendship proved to be especially beneficial to Tom's organization

Note: In January, 1998, this organization dedicated a new Educational Enrichment Center to Margaret's memory. In his comments that day, Tom Moen said:

"With Margaret's guidance, we raised over one million dollars in the past decade, including two successful capital campaigns. May Margaret's generous nature, desire to excel and caring attitude serve to inspire those who enter the Educational Enrichment Center."

Tom Moen, Madison, WI – a friend from the early '70s when he met Margaret and her first husband during a trip to Copenhagen

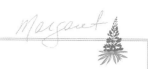

to Al and Rachael

$\mathscr{I}$am so very, very sorry for the loss of your wonderful
partner and mother. Margaret was a very generous, energetic
and positive person. She made a great difference in my life,
the lives of the people in our office and the lives of our clients
and students that she taught. She was a good friend!

It happened so quickly, and it is so hard to understand.
I hope that it is some consolation that she was able to finish
her dream of building your retirement life in northern
Wisconsin. Many people do not get the chance or do not take
the steps to realize their dreams. Al, what a loss that you
could not savor and enjoy this new phase in your life together
a little while longer. Rachael, I am sorry that you will not
be able to share your life,
as it unfolds in new and exciting directions, with your Mom.
It must feel so unfair. Margaret had too much to give, too
much energy, too much enthusiasm and too much love for her
participation in your life to be over now. I can truly picture
her in some new phase of her journey. In many ways
I am sure she will always be with you!

Neil Lerner, Madison, WI – a friend and professional colleague
at the Small Business Development Center

$\mathscr{I}$ took the dog for a long walk after your phone call. Temperature was in the 50s, semi cloudy, and the leaves were blowing. Why is it when death occurs your senses suddenly become so acutely aware of visions, sounds, smiles? And I keep asking myself why don't I make that happen every day? Margaret is in certainly a peaceful place; however, part of her will always remain at that beautiful house in the woods. I told the nurse who took care of her when she came to our OR, that she passed away, and he expressed the same feelings as I did. He, too, visits Bayfield on a regular basis.

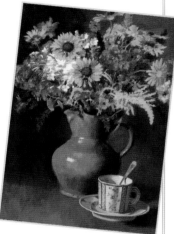

Finally, I also know the physical exhaustion that occurs when you care for a loved one in your home. I hope you will not feel guilty in just doing nothing for a bit, resting, and eating to restore your health. I know I lost 15 lbs. during those 4 months with my Mom. I thought this card truly represents what Margaret and you tried to portray with your guests.

Peg Maginnis, Madison, WI – a B&B guest in August, 1996 and a nurse at the hospital where Margaret received chemotherapy

*I*t is with great sadness and not a little shock that I heard
of Margaret's passing. Margaret was a very special woman.
She will live on in the memory of all of us whose lives she touched.
Her ability to teach, guide and create will be missed.
She was so excited by the Artesian House venture.
I'm glad she had the opportunity to start her dream
and saddened that she had so little time to enjoy it.

Sandra Jones, Madison, WI – a member of Margaret's
Cardinal Stritch MBA class

I wanted to be with you for the memorial service for Margaret.
Fortunately and unfortunately, I won't be able to do so.
Margaret is part of the reason why.
On November 2nd I'll be flying to Las Vegas to interview
for a position. Margaret's teaching, advising and being a great mentor
got me to this place. I cannot tell you how much she meant to me
as a teacher, mentor and friend. As you know she was quite the
woman. Our class respected and marvelled at how she did life!
Nothing was impossible; it all can be done – you just have to want
to, seemed to be her motto. I hurt and feel for all those who knew
her. Even more I feel for those who will never know her.
Her presence will remain a very special part of my life.

Maureen Fox, Las Vegas, NV – a member of the Cardinal Stritch MBA class

$\mathscr{O}$know that it has taken me a long time to write. To come to the reality that Margaret is gone, has taken a while. I want you to know some of the wonderful thoughts we have of her. First of all, she made the best coffee in the world. She had this old china drip coffee pot that she used which was the best! She could play bridge better than anyone I knew. We would get a babysitter for the kids and go for an afternoon of bridge. The best was when the girls were toddlers. We shared child care tips, recipes, stories and time together. Little did I know how precious that time would become.

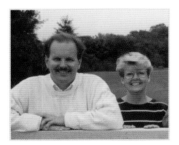

Dennis and Dianne VanLaningham

Whenever I think of Margaret I smile. She had the most beautiful smile of anyone in the world. She had a positive personality like no one else. She was a friend like no other I have ever had. There wasn't anything we couldn't share.

Dennis and Dianne, Manitowoc, WI
Best friends with Margaret and her first husband when all four lived in Manitowoc.
Both families had daughters the same age.

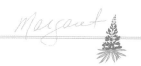

$\mathscr{I}$ m so very sorry about Margaret. I've tried to think of something I could say that might give you and your family even the slightest moment of comfort or peace. Yet every thought seems hollow, every expression trivial.

How many times have I heard "Life's not fair" and brushed it away as just another platitude? Sadly, that unexpected phone call this morning gave the words an unwelcome reality.

At an AA meeting yesterday, a man observed that any time we ask "Why did this happen to me?" we are casting ourself in the role of victim – a role I've never known you to assume. All that notwithstanding, it's impossible not to second guess a divine entity who would act in such a seemingly capricious manner. What I know for certain is that you and Margaret had some terrific years together. The almost tangible love and devotion flowing between the two of you at last summer's party made me ache with admiration and envy. So many people never even come close to achieving what you accomplished. We grieve at Margaret's leaving us all so soon, but still rejoice for the time you were able to share. Please know your family is in my heart and prayers. And don't ever forget: to live in hearts one leaves behind is not to die.

Claire Ortwein, Madison, WI – a colleague and friend of Al's
at the Hospital Association who knew Margaret

$\mathcal{D}$ear Margaret,

If I were in your shoes, I would want to know.
If I could walk with you, I'd want to let you hear.
There's so much more I'd have in store
For earth, for family, for my dear friends, for me.

What footprints will I leave
for those who want to walk with me?
Did I do enough, which path would I walk?
Whose hands would I hold, who would hold me?

I'd want to know that I meant so damned much
to those who shared my life. That I was truly loved.
That I showed you how to look at the winter with awe
and appreciate its infinite, pristine beauty.

Please tell me that you love me and you think about me
In the wildflowers, on the water, in my kitchen, at my table.
In the laughter, in the snow, in the forest, on the bike trail.
In front of the fire, in a look, with a hug and a kiss.

With all my love, Laura

Laura Sunday, Petaluma, CA – Al's sister-in-law;
she and Margaret enjoyed a special bond.

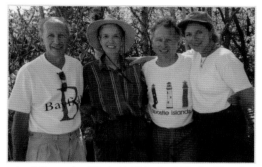

Margaret and Al camped and biked with Al's brother, Michael and his wife, Laura.
This was their final outing together, near Bayfield, in August, 1996.

Family holiday letter, December, 1996

𝒟ear Family & Friends. . . It's been a helluva year.

People write catching-up letters at the end of a year to send
to all those people who they're perennially out of touch with.
Normally it's too normal. But this year has been full of wake
up calls, bad news and some good news.

First the bad. Our family lost a truly cherished member,
Margaret Rdzak, my brother Al's dear wife and a woman who picked
up our family and moved it a few large degrees in a really wonderful
direction. I lost my dad a few years ago and felt it deeply, but
Margaret's battle with stomach cancer was a different kind of loss.
It took only a few months from diagnosis to her passing. It was
unimaginably fast, just really hard to understand. And Margaret,
along with her daughter, Rachael, and Al, demonstrated levels...

...of courage, fortitude and, ultimately, dignity
that were so heartening and heartbreaking all at once.
In the end, Margaret's closest kin and
a few friends kept a vigil at The Artesian House, finally bidding
goodbye and closing a chapter in all of our lives. She will be sorely
missed, and she leaves not only memories for us all, but a sense
of nobility you don't see but a few times in our lives.

*Michael Sunday, Petaluma, CA – Al's brother and Laura joined Margaret
and Al for biking and camping in Wisconsin, Minnesota and California.*

I have been wanting to write this note for months.
I heard about you and Margaret's decision to follow your dream
in Bayfield. Happiness is enjoying and appreciating each moment and
never looking back...no what if. *(Friend)* told me about Margaret's
death. All three of us had some great moments together.
I know you and Margaret were excited about your adventure
in Bayfield. I am sure you are wondering why bad things happen
to good people. The answer will come from Margaret in the messages
she sends to you each day for the rest of your life. Margaret is in a
better place to help herself and help you. We learn a lot in our
relationships we have in life. The last lesson is that
we are learning each day for a lifetime. So Margaret isn't gone.
She's with you in another way. . .still caring.

*Kevin Keighron, Prescott, AZ – a hospital executive in Wisconsin while
Al was with the Hospital Assn. who knew Margaret*

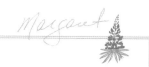

Written to Al

*N*o, we've never met, but I do want you to know how saddened I was to hear about Margaret's death. It seems far from fair that someone with so much to give would have her life interrupted in what should have been mid-stream. I had the distinct pleasure to work with Margaret in Madison. What I will always remember about her is her radiant smile, her enthusiasm for solving problems and her zestful approach towards life. In the brief time that I knew her, she left a mark on my own life. I do hope that you find comfort in knowing that Margaret's memory will continue to live in the hearts of those who knew her and whose lives she touched – and, believe me, like me, there are a lot of us out there!

Salli Martyniak, Madison, WI
Salli's words clearly came from the heart and reflected the feelings of many.

*T*hough I only knew Margaret for a short duration of time, she quickly became very special. Once again, I have been made aware of how vastly important each minute of our daily life is. I want to thank you, Al, for allowing me to help with Margaret's care. You and your family were a wonderful team to work with.

Carol L., Ashland, WI – a volunteer with Regional Hospice in Ashland
who provided care during Margaret's final two weeks

$\mathscr{I}$was shocked and deeply saddened to hear about Margaret.
I am so glad she called me last April when you were here
in Minneapolis. We talked for a good 45 minutes, catching
up on each other's lives. I gave her names for your mailing list
of other friends from the Copenhagen group that live
in the Twin Cities area.

I remember her telling me at our last reunion that you both
were going to start a B&B in Bayfield. I am so glad she got
to see the reality of that dream.

I am so sorry for your loss; she was far too young.
I will miss her.

Pattie, Minneapolis, MN – a friend of Margaret's
from the Copenhagen trip in the early '70s

$\mathscr{L}$ast week I went skiing at Winter Park, huffing and puffing
around the Base Loop and on to NoseDive. I thought about you
and Margaret being there with me, and I stopped on one of the
hills and thought of Margaret's spirit going home and how
fortunate I was to have known her on this earth.

Tomorrow, Saturday, is the darkest, the winter solstice,
which now gives way to light, a little at a time.

Carol Bohn, Lac du Flambeau, WI – a colleague of Margaret's in Kenosha in the '80s;
now an artist in northern Wisconsin whose work hangs at the B&B

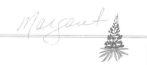

That I am writing on Margaret's birthday (*December 7*) adds poignancy to my thoughts. "Life is a journey" says the prayer book, "and death a destination." Margaret's journey was full of energy and enthusiasm for her work and full of love for you and Rachael. It all ended too soon. I hope that memories of happier times can ease the sadness and loneliness you feel. Please know that Margaret is remembered with affection and respect.

Betsy Brown, Kenosha, WI – friend and colleague while Margaret was in Kenosha;
also a friend of Al's

November 20, 1996
Written to Margaret, not knowing she had died

Thank you so much for the lovely note you sent me when you returned my deposit check for a stay at The Artesian House. As you may recall, I had to cancel our stay because I was diagnosed with breast cancer and was scheduled for a mastectomy. Your words about your own struggle with stomach cancer and the healing powers of The Artesian House and its surroundings couldn't have come at a better time for me. Thank you for those words, and I wish you continued strength. I look forward to re-scheduling our visit to The Artesian House and to thanking you in person for your taking the time to send me such encouraging words.

Marjorie Smelstor, Altoona, WI
Margaret was deeply concerned over Marjorie's need to cancel her reservation.
They never met.

$\mathcal{I}$ just heard of Margaret's death.

I'm truly sorry for your loss. My husband died 2 1/2 years ago.
As hard as it was to see his decline, we both treasured that time
together. We were ready to say goodbye and let go.

It was a relief to know he was released from his tormented body.

We will always miss our loved ones. Good memories help to get
through each day. I'm sure Margaret must have felt satisfaction in
seeing dreams of your B&B become a reality.

Judy, Grand View, WI – proprietor of a B&B in northern Wisconsin;
first met Margaret in June, 1996 at a regional B&B meeting

Margaret

Rather than mourn...

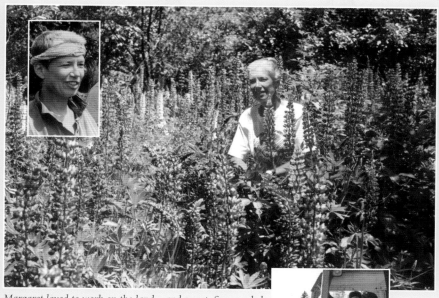

Margaret loved to work on the land... and sweat. Surrounded, at The Artesian House, by the lupines she loved.

At The Wilson Street Grill, our favorite restaurant in Madison.

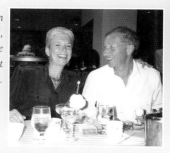

With classes, clients or heavy equipment, she was in control.

*At right: Margaret and Rachael
catch up on some
mother-daughter stuff.*

*Below: the same,
but a few years earlier.*

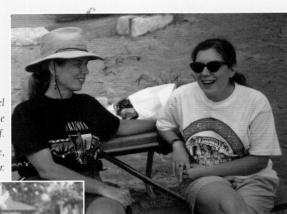

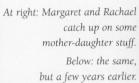

Sun, wind and a smile.

*Kayaking near Bayfield just after
her first chemotherapy.*

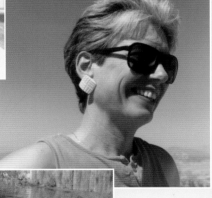

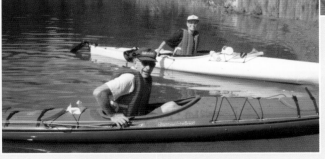

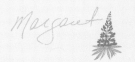

...the absence of the flame

At right: with Al in Door County.
Below: enjoying the sound of a rushing river in West Virginia.

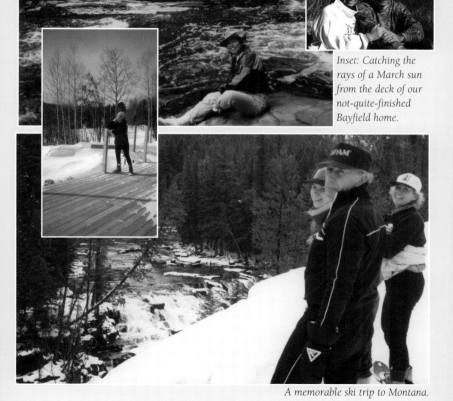

Inset: Catching the rays of a March sun from the deck of our not-quite-finished Bayfield home.

A memorable ski trip to Montana.

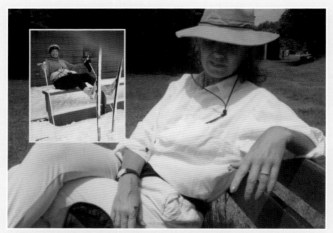

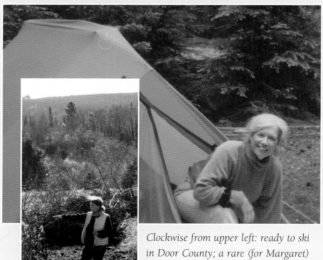

Clockwise from upper left: ready to ski in Door County; a rare (for Margaret) quiet moment; emerging from a night of camping; inspecting our land in Bayfield.

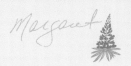

Margaret

let us celebrate...

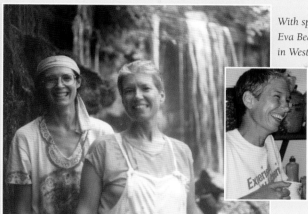

With spiritual soul mate
Eva Bear-Johnson
in West Virginia.

Margaret +
coffee = smile!

Cooking with Eva's daughter, Mir.

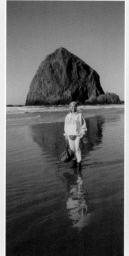

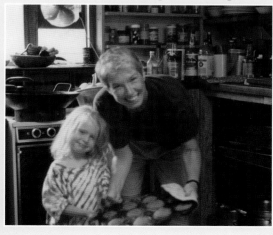

On the beach near Seattle.

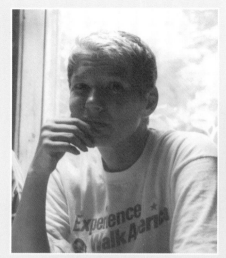

The way many saw her in meetings —
thoughtful, attentive, focused.

Ready for a winter beach
party in Milwaukee.

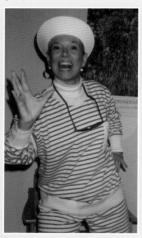

Equally comfortable
modeling a new gift,
or, below, enjoying
a winter picnic.

Above: our only photo
of Margaret in the
B&B kitchen.

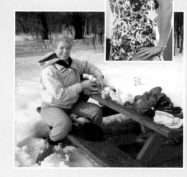

At home in Madison.

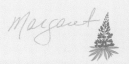

Margaret

...how brightly it burned.

Three generations: her mother, Rachael, and Margaret compare smiles. Below: showing off a new hat.

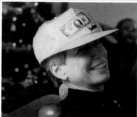

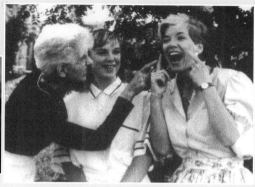

Left: with Al in Boston. Below: in the woods in her favorite hat... perhaps looking to the future.

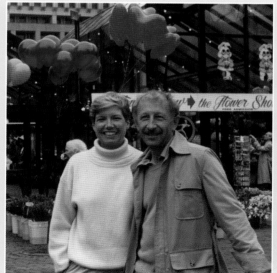

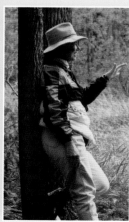

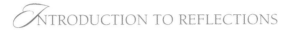

$\mathcal{I}$NTRODUCTION TO REFLECTIONS

$\mathcal{A}$ small group of people who knew Margaret
in vastly different ways were invited to write their
thoughts for this section.

They include: family, friends, professional colleagues,
guests at The Artesian House and a few who quite
likely never would have met her
had it not been for her illness.

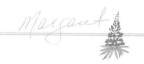

REFLECTIONS

*D*ear Margaret,

I feel sad – angry. Angry because we only had a relationship
for such a short time before you died. Yes we are sisters –
me being older – but in so many ways you were older and more

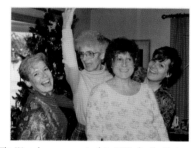

The Weyenberg women at a late 1980s family Christmas
From left: Margaret, their mother, Mae, Kathy and Trisha

mature than I was. It took me so many years – too many –
to realize how special you were. Before I was able to look at you and
your ways as healthy, nurturing, giving. I guess "sister stuff" – "family
stuff" got in the way. I had such tunnel vision. I'm angry it took so
long before my love for my sister was a true love – unconditional
love. Before I was grown up enough to know it was O.K. to be
outspoken – to know what you wanted in life and to go for it with...

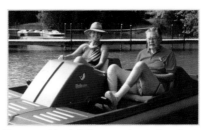

Margaret and her dad, George, navigate in Door County.

...GUSTO! You scared me, Margaret. Your zest scared me. Your persistence scared me. Oh! how long it took me to get to that point. That's why I'm angry. When my blinders came off – oh! the things I learned from my little sister. The joy of having a relationship with you. To finally know the real you. Not to be afraid anymore of a relationship with you. How sad and unfair – it was so short. I don't begin to understand the ways of Spirit. Why wasn't our journey allowed to go into Old Age? I'm grateful for what was. Grateful for the gifts of emotions I've had and continue to have because you are my sister – Anger, Sadness, Joy, Frustration! And, Margaret, I'll be forever grateful for you giving me the gift of your dying and death. You showed me I will have nothing to fear; that it can be a beautiful experience. They say memories are what keep a person's spirit alive. What a symphony of memories I have. And last but not least, Margaret, the smile that comes to my soul when I think of how much more interesting eternity must be for God since you are back. Love, Kathy

Kathy Lux, Kimberly, WI – Margaret's older sister; works in health care;
Margaret took special joy in watching Kathy bloom, personally and professionally.

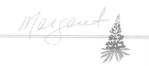

𝑀argaret . . .

Thank you for those eight days you gave me.
The phone call. . ."Come now, Trisha. I want you to come now."
Kathy and I driving around that last curve on a brilliant
Sunday until I see for the first time the magnificent house
you and Al built in the northern Wisconsin hills.

Eight days left to be with you, to help you, to know and love my
sister. And, as sisters go, we had our differences, our never
expressed competitiveness – you be the smart one – I'll be the
artsy one. The walls that siblings build were there. But in those
eight days you let us all in. I got to know my sister that I had
missed for many years and was sorry for that . . .but so grateful
that you let us take care of you and let us be part of your
incredible journey. I love you.

Trisha Weyenberg-Lipson, Tarrytown, NY
Margaret's younger sister; works in publishing in New York City. She has a marvellous voice
and sang "The Irish Blessing" at Margaret's Memorial Service in Madison.

𝒯hree years ago, I shared these words with family and friends
who gathered at Margaret's memorial service in celebration of her
life. As I re-read these words, I'm struck by how I wouldn't
change a word. Because Margaret was the most genuine person
I ever knew, the pictures painted by the words of this book are...

...enduring and will continue to ring true in our hearts
as we remember.

Where do I stop? Where do I start?

It's a privilege to be here to celebrate Margaret in our lives – to share memories of a woman who loved intensely, who lived life with such zest, who made a significant difference in so many lives.

Margaret, I know you're here tonight. Your spirit is with us. You are still a part of us and, kiddo, you wouldn't miss an incredible party like this! So, my dear friend, here I go.

It's impossible to fully capture Margaret in words, but some thoughts come quickly to mind. First, a visible picture flashes by – one of beauty: big brown eyes, dazzling smile and animated features and gestures. She lit up a room when she walked in, and we were glad to be in that room. But there is more, much more than physical beauty. Words come to mind . . .words that Margaret would say are "too much," but this is one of those few times when she isn't in control.

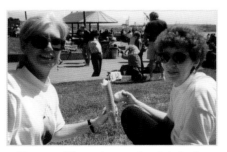

Margaret and Karen enjoy sun and snacks in Seattle.

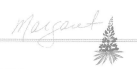

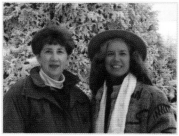

Amazing, opinionated, full of grace, bright, enthusiastic, wise, confident, loving, witty, generous. A woman of remarkable depth, indomitable spirit, high standards, passion for people and causes . . . a community and family builder who brought people together. Full of fun/out for adventure. A classy woman with just the right amount of sassiness stirred in for good measure!

Margaret was an extraordinary presence. In her presence, we came face-to-face with a genuine person, a person who knew herself, who let us know her and who encouraged us to know ourselves. She told me at times that she thought she might be "found out" – that Rachael, her daughter, might realize that she wasn't "wonder mother." But the truth is that Margaret was so open that we did know her. We knew her limitations as well as her strengths. . . and we knew how fortunate we were to be in her presence.

Margaret followed her bliss. She made choices to act on what she knew to be true. Not only did she know how to pinch pennies...

...with the best of them, but she also knew how to pinch more life out of each moment than anyone I ever knew. She lived life to the hilt. She acted on her passions...even when it meant struggles with physical limitations or too many priorities and demands. A friend once described her as a comet – one who sometimes left "debris" in her path! Her gifts were many and extraordinary. She used them as fully as anyone could in almost 50 years of life. We were beneficiaries of those gifts. She saw more clearly (even on dark days) than most of us will in our lifetimes. We relied on her sound judgement because she knew what was needed in a situation, saw options and knew which were best and could put a puzzle together (whether on a table or in real life).

Margaret made a difference in so many of our lives. Many have shared with Al how she was a mentor and friend to them – a guide and a counselor. I have the picture of someone who calls from further up the mountain and says – "Come on up. The view is wonderful. Watch the rocks. Stay on the path when you can – or if you can't, OK, you'll make it up safely."

Margaret saw what was needed for us to achieve our dreams. She listened to us, nudged us gently and not-so-gently. Sometimes pushed, encouraged, affirmed, nurtured us, provided us with a model, held us accountable and helped us grow.

Margaret was the best of friends, and she loved her family deeply. She was there in the good times and the hard times. We could

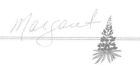

count on Margaret. She accepted us, loved us.
She told us the truth – gently (and not so gently, when needed).
She was generous of spirit and time.

It is important that each of you – Margaret's family and friends –
are celebrated tonight. She did not become "Margaret" alone, and
recognized this. I was fortunate to have good conversations with her
almost daily. I wish I could share some of the stories about what
a difference you made in her life ... how much she needed you for
love and support. You helped to mold who she was. You let her be
Margaret. She drew from your strengths, your laughter, your good
times together. You enriched her with your presence and gifts.
She admired and loved you.

And finally, Margaret, none of us is prepared to say good-bye. Like
all of you, it's deeply sad for me not to have her presence in my life.
We can, though, be thankful for the time and memories we cherish.
Margaret said she planned to see us again. That's our plan too.

Right after she was diagnosed, Margaret told me, "You know, Karen,
I will be healed – whether it is in this life or the next."
We trust these words and are comforted. We miss you deeply,
Margaret. You are in our hearts forever, We love you.
Good-bye for now.

Karen Julesberg, Madison, WI
Karen and Margaret's lives crossed through work, and their close friendship –
enhanced by coffee and conversation and shared vacations – developed into one of deep mutual
trust, love and understanding.

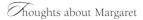
*T*houghts about Margaret

Margaret Rdzak traveled through life at the side of her friends.
Sometimes she was right there next to you
and sometimes out of sight,
but always traveling with you.
When you came to a fork in the road,
she had a way of appearing.
She never said which fork to take, but she
asked the pointed questions which revealed the right course.
Often it would be an opportunity never previously explored.
Usually, it would require a larger leap than you
had anticipated or hoped for.

When the path became a freeway and life passed in a blur,
she would slow the process down, and suddenly balance, humor
and joy would be restored. Margaret had special clarity
on life that few exhibit or express. Time spent with Margaret
was a shot of renewal.
Often, in times of reflection, the question,
"What would Margaret say?"
brings that sense of direction and clarity.
She taught her friends well.

Nan Zimdars, Madison, WI
a professional colleague, sailing partner, financial advisor
and the "great boss" referred to in the top letter on page 25

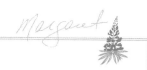

$\mathcal{D}$ear Margaret,

I hardly had time to know you. We met late in 1994, two short years before you left this world. I remember a vivacious, strikingly beautiful woman who came as a consultant to help my community. I soon came to know you as a multi-faceted, highly imaginative person. Your great skills as a communicator impressed me. You not only used the right language, you were able to break with protocol to cause us to think. And you were a great listener, hearing and understanding our feelings and fears, not just our words. I liked your wildness, Margaret – the wildness of a bird in flight, a rushing river, a deer in the field. You had a certain reverence for life which came from having lived life and having dealt with its ups and downs. You were alive to living.

I respected your keen perception of reality as it was. You could handle tough things. You looked at our community and said, "Okay, here are religious women with a vision outside the box. I will help you pull the cart up the hill." You hooked on with us; gave us energy. You made it feel like there were 10,000 people working with us, while all the time it was just one Margaret. You were a religious person in the sense you knew you were a creature of and had a reverence for God. I had the sense that you talked to God across the table, saw God in many different ways. You weren't limited by church or God-talk. God was bigger than that, and yet you respected us as sisters. Some days I watch a...

...red-tailed hawk gliding overhead. Margaret, you could glide so easily! Many times I feel your presence as you keep watch over us.

Mary David Walgenbach, OSB, Prioress – Sisters of Saint Benedict, Madison, WI
Sr. Mary David was a client and friend as Margaret worked with the sisters to create a unique ecumenical community near Madison.

September, 1999

$\mathscr{I}$ am one of the luckiest people I know. I was with Margaret during her last days, when she gave us the greatest gift on earth, and let us see a piece of heaven. I watched in wonder as a smile of pure joy came across her face as she spoke with her mother and others, whom she had loved and lost, as she traveled to their world. I was amazed when Margaret spoke of beautiful music she heard even though the room was silent. Margaret would close her eyes and travel between conversations, asking questions *there* and still answering our questions *here*. She told us that she could only tell us a little bit about the place she visited because that was *their* rules. Now I know with all my heart that there is a heaven and that it is beautiful. This message gives me great peace, knowing that I will someday see my sister Martha again. I also know that Margaret carried my message of love to Martha. As my daughters, Lucy and Sonya, grow up and ask me if heaven exists, I can share the story of their Grandma Margaret. And when they ask me if there really are angels, I can honestly tell them, "Yes, Margaret told me so."

Sara Chechik, Minneapolis, MN
Sara is the wife of Al's youngest son, Joel. Despite a 19-year age difference, she and Margaret built a very special relationship – perhaps partly mother-daughter and partly as sisters.

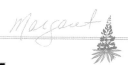

Margaret

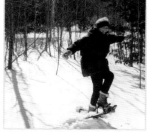

*W*ings

Hair flying, feet flying, Margaret
on skis, Margaret in snowshoes, Skis
skim, shoes crunch, arms stretch, air
embraces. Smile wide, wide as arms, beckon
us, draws us in.
Sun shines, sun embraces, holds
Margaret, draws her up. Clouds split,
she slips through, we cry, she is gone.
She is gone, but she is here, slipping
through sleeping clouds, skimming
snow, touching earth, embracing us
until we fly, sneaking through split clouds.
We cry.
She is here.

Marjorie Audette, St. Paul, MN
For several years, Marge and her husband, Gene, shared a January week – plus wine
and conversation – with Margaret and Al at a northern Wisconsin timeshare.

$\mathcal{M}$y first visit with Margaret was at her request.
Hospital room and hospital gown notwithstanding, Margaret
was a striking presence. Not in the least arrogant or aloof,
Margaret had a respect for herself that made her invitation a privilege.
Margaret also struck me as a woman of courage.
Very early in our conversation, it was clear that she wanted to go deep.
No platitudes, no formulas. Her keen mind freed her doubts and fears
straight on. Together we traced her spiritual heritage, took stock
of the meaning of her life and her choices, made preparations for the
dying she knew was not far off. Margaret seemed to trust our time
together, and I respected her candid openness.
Margaret and her husband, Al, also gave me a gift I rarely receive.
As a hospital chaplain, most of my work takes place in institutional
settings. Margaret and Al invited me into their home. There, in this place
that had been their shared dream, we shared the closing of Margaret's life.
Later, I had the privilege of leading a memorial service for Margaret,
again amidst the beauty of her north country home.
Even though our time together was brief, Margaret made a lasting
impression on me. Two, perhaps three other times in my fifteen years
of ministry, have I encountered people who were so intentional in their
spiritual and relational preparations for leaving this life.
Margaret was a woman of strength and beauty, courage and intellect.
I miss her.

Kent Seldal, Hospital Director of Pastoral Care, Washburn, WI
Kent was a source of support and assistance for everyone who gathered
at our home during Margaret's final days.

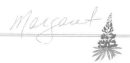

*𝒯*houghts of Margaret Rdzak

The smile. The image that comes to mind when I think of Margaret is her smile. Our first encounter was at an open house we held here at Pinehurst Inn – an opportunity to meet other innkeepers and show them our place and work. Margaret came into the kitchen with this wonderful, broad smile, recognizing that we were on the same path to starting a venture as innkeepers. I immediately appreciated this woman who carried with her a strong spirit and presence.

The connections. There are often connections when getting to know a person. There seemed to be an instant understanding of our mutual respect – indeed, passion – for Bayfield and the Chequamegon Bay area. There was an instant recognition, although unspoken, of the joy we anticipated in sharing this with guests in our respective bed & breakfasts. Our dreams were on similar paths.

The spirit. Margaret had an aura about her. Through the summer of her illness, I often thought about how much I wanted to get to know her better. I knew this woman had a spirit about her that I could learn much from. I treasured the bits of time we spent together. The brief visits as her illness progressed provided a unique view of this spirit, for Margaret reached a place of peace with her impending death. She knew she had lived well. Her spirit carries on inside the lovely house, and in the fields and woods.

Nancy Sandstrom, Bayfield, WI
Nancy and her husband, Steve, own a B&B close to The Artesian House. They began their adventure as new innkeepers in the spring of 1996, just as Margaret and I were beginning ours.

*A*fter several years of knowing about Margaret, I, at last, got to know her. She struck me as a "no bullshit," yet gentle woman who believed that sincerity of soul was the true measure of a person. Only after I accepted her in my life did I realize the genuineness and purity of her soul. Before she died, we reached a peace. My only regret is that I hadn't pursued that peace far sooner. Perhaps then I could have shared more than a glimmer of her happiness, spontaneity and warmth.

Marc Chechik, St. Louis, MO
Marc is Al's oldest son. He and Margaret had a relationship that was initially tenuous, but in her final days became mutually understanding and accepting.

*M*argaret... . to me

The little I know about Margaret comes from three sources . . . the brief conversations with her family and friends at the memorial service, the look in your eyes, Al, when her name is spoken, and the time I have spent at The Artesian House feeling her presence.

The way I picture Margaret, she was a woman who had passion. . . passion for every single adventure she decided to wrap her arms around. She was a woman's woman. A woman who didn't let the roadblocks of life cause her to blink, even for an instant. A woman whose depth and spirit was so rich that it continues to live on in every life that she touched. She was a true messenger of integrity and rightness. A woman we might call "stern,"

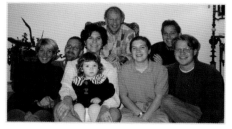

*Front row, from left: Sara Chechik with Lucy (the only grandchild Margaret
was able to meet) Rachael; Carl Mickelson. Back row, from left: Victoria
and Marc Chechik; Al; Sara's husband, Joel.*

but who was tender as dew. The perfect combination of strength

and humility. The reason I know this is because, in Margaret,

I see the memory of my grandmother (who died December 6, 1997).

These women are rare.

It's such a shame the world continues on without them.

Victoria Hatfield Chechik, St. Louis, MO
*Vicki is Marc's wife. She never met Margaret, so her perceptions, as she says,
are second and third-hand — but no less vivid, clear and dead-on.*

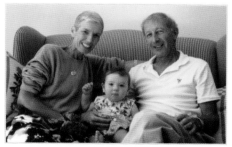

Margaret with Lucy and Al, August, 1996

$\mathscr{R}$emembering Margaret

I feel sad when I think of Margaret's death. I also experience happiness and comfort when I recall the wonderful opportunity of enjoying her as a professional colleague and dear friend.

These adjectives describe Margaret in my thoughts: dynamic, energetic, enthusiastic, zealous, sincere, stimulating, courageous in adversity, optimistic, futuristic, generous, loving, respectful and charitable. I recollect her affection and devotion toward her husband, daughter and parents. Margaret will live on in my memories as a very special person.

Dolores Olson, Charlotte, N.C.
Although she was about a generation older than Margaret, I believe Dolores
found her a good sounding board – perhaps not unlike a daughter
who can offer an ear for listening, a shoulder when needed.

$\mathscr{D}$ear Margaret,

How I miss you! On cold rainy days such as this, you were always the sunshine that would light up a room. You had a way about you that could enhance anyone in a room once you entered. I always think of you as a brilliant swath of Red through an otherwise neutral world. I am so lucky to have known you.

In the early part of our friendship, I was in awe of the power you appeared to carry. You stood up for me at work, without asking

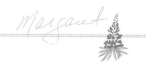

me, for months when I was trying to deal with a difficult pregnancy. You helped me to see what it meant to stand up for and respect yourself in the face of adversity. Numerous pep talks cemented our relationship. Throughout the years, you were always there when I needed you, especially with Nicholas. You should see him now; you would be so proud!

I think you do.

You helped me to find balance in my life between work and family, and, most importantly within myself. The days you taught me to sail still give me such peace to remember them. Taking an afternoon off to glide across the lake filled us with exhilaration and inner energy. It cleared the cobwebs and helped us to find peace in our busy lives. I haven't sailed since, but I will someday. I am not yet willing to dilute those memories.

I think you understand.

You gave me a good awareness to nurturing and raising a child. Many of us have part of this innately, but the ability to probe into the root of behaviors was something you excelled in. This has helped me tremendously with my little Margaret. Did you know that she has a smile that shines like yours and such sparkly eyes?

I think you do.

You gave to me so freely, and so much of that continues on that you are regularly in my thoughts. I often sit back and try to. . .

. . .think how you would approach an issue, and it really helps.
I hope I gave to you even a fraction of what you gave to me.
As I go through my days, and feel the brush of your angel wings on
my cheek, I am comforted. But oh, how I miss you!
I think you understand.

Love, Margy Acker, Madison, WI
Margy became very close as a colleague and a friend when she and Margaret
worked together at Smith & Gesteland and later when both pursued other dreams.

I met Margaret and Al in what was Margaret's 49th year.
Our friendship was fairly short, but seemed to carry with it a
lifetime of intuition and understanding. I had, what I considered,
the honor to be a part of finishing (or starting) a dream they shared.
My trade is interior design, and the dream I speak of is The Artesian
House. I operate my business solely based on the "hearts" of those I
work with, not on the money I'm able to make on the project. This
mindset was what excited me so much about Margaret. I felt I had
met a woman who could almost look into your soul, if you would
let her, and was happy to give just as much back. This, in my
opinion, is a rare gift in anyone's life. It's a hard thing to bare who
you are as an individual . . .It's precious to find those that know
without having to tell them. I will never forget you, Margaret.

Deb Casey, Washburn, WI
Deb came into our lives as an interior designer and became a close friend.
She and Margaret bonded – quickly and deeply.

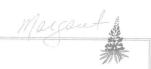

$\mathcal{D}$ear Margaret,

The progress of my thoughts is coming along slowly,
as do many of my projects. As the ground that is soon
to be broken has never seen light or metal of the steel shovel;
it is yet untouched. God said, out of the earth I will create man –
in his image, the image of God. There has never been, or ever
will be, a greater architect or builder than God. There is no greater
joy than to know God. Not me, not you, or anything else
is in total control. That all of God's projects are completed
on time and are perfectly done, without flaw.

There are no call backs.

The door will always open.

Margaret, in our eyes the years were cut far too short,
but the master builder had completed his project, and what
He left behind was not anything human hands could have made.
Thank you for reaching down and touching all of us –
and especially me.

Gregory S. Carrier, Bayfield, WI
Greg and his company built the B&B. He answered our questions,
helped solve problems and became a friend. He said we'd open a year
after we broke ground, June 15, 1995.
We opened June 14, 1996.

*S*ometimes

Sometimes life gives
the gift
of a conversation
to be remembered.

I had two with Margaret.

A nurse, who attended my son's birth,
now attended Margaret's dying.
She said Margaret was a woman
of spiritual wonderings and it would be
good for me, from hospice, to meet her.

In a summer hospital room I met her.
She talked for an hour or more about illness
and desire and life and yearning and love
and friends and family and death and earth.
She sought guidance from within the clarity of her heart.
Her eyes spoke with passionate loveliness.
She needed to know
what was important to be/do/finish in her life-too-short.
Although I went as the helper-guy,
I left knowing she was the teacher.
I was full and smiled from the inside.

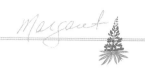

And the second was near her life's end
at the B&B.
The words were few.
She asked for wisdom.
I said, "Trust"

& gave a Superior stone.
Then waited while she slept
As the clock ticked minutes into hours
And Al erranded.

All the way home
the image of her
strength and weakness,
her wisdom and wonderment
her peacefulness and her angst
visited me.

And, she visits still.

Phil Garrison, Duluth, MN
Phil was director of Regional Hospice in Ashland when we first contacted that organization.
He and the Hospice staff and volunteers gave genuine meaning to the hospice goal
of providing quality of life – for patient and family.

A Shining Star

I first got to know Margaret, or so I thought, when I interviewed her for the marketing director position at Smith & Gesteland LLP, Certified Public Accountants, where I was the managing partner. At lunch we discovered that we had traveled together on the same University of Wisconsin System-sponsored trip to the former Soviet Union in the late '60s. Margaret was the consummate interviewee. Her poise, enthusiasm, genuine interest and passion for her profession were apparent and grew more evident each day we worked together. Margaret, in her new position, was responsible for the development of a marketing department – new territory for a very traditional CPA firm. She thrived on new challenges and always put her whole being into the task at hand. Her signature on the development of the marketing program and in the firm's strategic planning initiatives is still obvious today. Prodding us stodgy CPA types to think a new way was a job she relished.Thanks, Margaret, for getting us on the right road.

Margaret's sense of humor was evident every day. She always (well, almost always) had a smile on her face. That enthusiasm and attitude was responsible for helping me to look at my profession in a new light and not take it quite so seriously.

I will never forget when Margaret and I arrived midweek at a resort location in south central Wisconsin to prepare

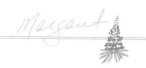

for a firm planning session beginning the next day. We came upon
a group of elderly ladies leaving the main dining room. At first
glance, many of these faces looked somewhat familiar to me.
I thought nothing more of it until it appeared that most everyone
in the group was intently watching us and whispering, not so
discretely, to each other.

The "buzz" of the group turned out to be gossip as to how to
tell one of their fellow church members, my Mom, that her son was
wandering around the resort, midweek, with a woman who was
not his wife. Thankfully, my Mom came forward from the group,
and I was able to introduce her to Margaret, thus dispelling
the rumor of infidelity. Thereafter, Margaret often enjoyed bringing
up her role as the "other woman."

I will always remember Margaret's zest for life, her humor,
her hard work, her enthusiasm and the strong relationships
she developed with many diverse people. I will treasure her
friendship always. From the red-jeweled stars over the Kremlin
in Moscow to the clear, bright stars over Lake Superior,
I will never forget this shining star.

Chuck Gietzel, Madison, WI
Chuck was Margaret's boss when she joined Smith & Gesteland in the newly-created position
of marketing director. I'm not sure either knew where the road would lead.
It led to a solid friendship – professional and personal.

Memories of Margaret

I first met Margaret when I joined the staff of Kenosha Memorial Hospital as the Nurse Recruiter in 1979. Margaret had been hired just shortly before this time as the Public Relations Manager.

I was 26, Margaret was 33. I recall my boss suggesting that Margaret and I should get to know each other. In his affable and always kind (but sometimes too naive) way, he saw our similarities. I, however, the socially backward one and not much for pleasantries of unfocused social interaction, saw only the vast differences between Margaret's natural style and mine.

I was prepared to be rebuffed, as I had been frequently by the "in crowd" during my schooling.

But Margaret did not rebuff me. Yes, she had been part of the "in crowd" in high school as I would later learn. But she had also experienced being an outcast from that same crowd for voicing her values, so she could empathize with my past.

She was married when I met her – with a 5-year-old little girl, Rachael. But that was to change soon. As would both of our lives.

Over the next 17 years, Margaret and I shared a variety of experiences that would cause our lives – personal and professional – to intersect in life-altering ways. We would both see the end of the marriages that existed when we met . . .we would both lose our mothers, and I, my father as well . . .we would

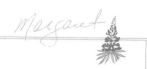

become close working colleagues as the hospital became
embroiled in three successive, physically and mentally challenging
and exhausting union organizing campaigns,
all of which the hospital won. . .we would collaborate in starting
a Management Women's support group to enable female leaders
at the hospital to accelerate their own leadership development.
Looking back, I realize that Margaret was a particular source
of power and positive outlook that sustained our group through
this period. . .Margaret and I shared one special benefit of
our roles in those union campaigns: the hospital's support while
we pursued our MBAs from the Executive Curriculum Program
at the University of Wisconsin at Milwaukee, both graduating
in 1984. . .we would both find a wonderful second marriage –
Margaret with Al Chechik in 1985, and I with Jim Clerc,
who would become my husband in Spring, 1995. It was Margaret
who offered two of the most meaningful readings at our wedding.
At the time of my wedding, Margaret and Al were in the midst
of planning their Bed and Breakfast in Bayfield, Wisconsin.
The spring of 1996 found Margaret supervising the construction
of the B&B. During that time she began to lose weight – by July
her weight loss prompted a visit to the doctor. Stomach cancer.

I saw Margaret one last time on a marvelous October weekend
at the B&B in Bayfield. She was a mere shadow of her former self...

...She was bedridden, although she was able to get up into a wheelchair. Hospice was providing care. Al, Rachael, Carl, Margaret's sisters Kathy and Trisha, Karen Julesberg, Al's sons Marc and Joel and Joel's wife Sara and 11-month old daughter Lucy were all there. The weather was glorious.

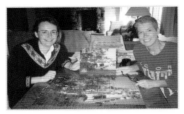

Margaret and Marilyn Clerc, after completing one of their easier puzzles. Union campaigns proved more challenging.

Margaret knew she did not have long to live.

We celebrated Al's 62nd birthday. We played with the baby. We tried to comfort one another and find meaning in the tragedy that was taking place. We took walks to try to maintain our composure around Margaret.

Margaret was one of the most positive influences over my life. She was consistently positive, upbeat, centered and grounded in a gracious type of interactive style that was uniquely her own. She fit the description of one who never met a stranger. She was highly principled and maintained that high level of expectation with all those around her. She invented patient and customer satisfaction before it became the "vogue." She epitomized the philosophy that

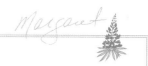

one must take risks if one is to be the person one deeply
desires to be. Margaret personified the saying "no guts, no glory,"
for she had adequate intestinal fortitude for all of us.

I still miss her terribly. I cannot seem to find another human
being who has the same combination of intellect, understanding,
gutsy pushiness, and inquisitiveness all combined into one.
I don't dwell on it – because I also learned from her that to dwell
on only sadness and loss is to rob your life of the joy that the
present can produce. I can only say thank you for the opportunity
of having known her and being blessed to become her friend.

I will always remember Margaret.

Marilyn Clerc, Columbus, IN
I can't expand on Marilyn's words. She and Margaret were linked for 17 years –
almost one-third of Margaret's life.

Margaret Rdzak

Margaret, I wish you were here to draft this for me.
I relied on you so much as we grew up together in Kenosha
at Kenosha Memorial Hospital. We were both motivated and rose
to the many challenges. I relied heavily on your writing ability
and advice. You were always strong, motivated and direct,
but also caring and with a wonderful smile on your face...

...We grew up together as professional colleagues ... and friends. If we had only been professional colleagues, you certainly would not have been so bold as to tell me I wore my ties too short, and that I needed to look more presentable for pictures. For you and me. . .and many others you worked with at Kenosha Memorial, it was a Camelot experience. God bless you and keep you.

John McGinty, Columbus, IN

As CEO at Kenosha Memorial Hospital, John was blessed with a strong group of women – Margaret was one – who worked actively to blend the achievement of hospital goals with their own professional development. To his credit, he gave them plenty of leeway!

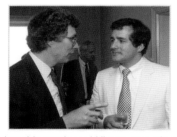

The authors of the preceding and following pieces, John McGinty, right, and Paul Ihlenfeld, at Margaret and Al's wedding in 1985.

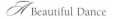

$\mathscr{A}$ Beautiful Dance

With the passing of time, my memories of Margaret have distilled into a moving collage of "integrated opposites."

I remember her as both powerful, bold and intense,

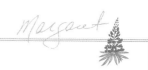

yet also,
keenly sensitive and, at times, fragile;

I remember her as both
committed to high standards and integrity,
yet also,
frequently the first to speak with compassion
or kindness for people whose weaknesses were
showing;

I remember her as both
wise and serious,

yet also,

a regular instigator of foolishness and fun.

For most, these opposites can't dance comfortably
together until old age, if then. For Margaret, not
only did the gift of this dance come early, but with
it, the capacity to help others to dance with her.

May her memory keep you dancing!

Paul Ihlenfeld, Hartland, WI
Paul was a long-time professional colleague and friend of Margaret's.
He performed Margaret and Al's wedding in 1985 and Margaret's memorial service
in Madison, November 2, 1996.

$\mathcal{W}$est Virginia, combined with our visit to Washington, D.C., will never go away as a turning point for me. Margaret invited me to join her for a week of volunteering at Gesundheit *(Note: Gesundheit is a proposed health care community in West Virginia referred to in the movie "Patch Adams")*. She had spent the major portion of her summer there – I, however, was hoping for a break from work at St. Joseph's *(hospital in San Diego, CA)*.

We met in Washington, D.C. and stayed over to visit the Vietnam War Memorial and see the sights. The memory of Margaret at the War Memorial as she searched for her past was so honest and moving. It was a sad time, but a special time as she acknowledged how life moves on – in wonderful ways.

Then we travelled to West Virginia through the hill country to Gesundheit where she was volunteering. For a westerner, it was wonderful, green and wild country marked by poverty. Margaret oriented me to the philosophy of Gesundheit – and it was a glorious purpose: to provide healthcare to all, regardless of ability to pay, at no cost – only contributions.

With Margaret, during the week, we took turns cooking our communal meals; doing back-breaking work in the garden; and taking breaks only to skinny dip in the ICE COLD lake on site. We also had a chance to participate in a sweat lodge one night.

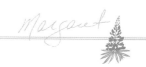

I thought I would suffocate, however, Margaret, as always, enjoyed the opportunity to experience the heat of the lodge too. My muscles were screaming, but Margaret was the "ever-ready bunny". One day our work detail was assigned to build a handicapped trail that would lead into the mountain. About 20 of us labored with shovels and pick axes to cut that trail. During our work, one of the foreign students working with us hit a beehive with his pick axe. With a swarm of bees chasing us, we tumbled pell-mell down the trail and did not stop until we were all in the ICE cold water of the lake – freezing, laughing, dirty and cold.

To get into the mountains, we decided that Margaret and I, plus a couple of volunteers, would

Whether swinging like kids or doing the "tourist thing" in D.C., Judy and Margaret had fun.

sleep on top of one of the mountains overnight in order to see the sun rise over the Blue Ridge. After working all day, four of us hiked up a mountain in the dark with one of the volunteers who knew the area. We had to keep a fire going all night to ward off the critters so we took turns on watch. We sang, we laughed, we told stories, we – sort of – slept. We were all awake just before dawn – mostly from sleeping on the hard, cold, wet ground...

...AND THE SUN CAME UP GLORIOUSLY. It was a sight I will never forget. We all were so quiet; I know I prayed my thanks for having the opportunity to see that sunrise and to welcome a new day in a very special way. I would never have gone if Margaret had not wanted to. She did so much to touch my life.

In that week I spent with her working as a volunteer, I learned so much about myself, thanks to Margaret. It was a time of giving back to others – and a chance to enjoy a simple life with a wonderful friend. I have not been able to see the movie *(Patch Adams)* because I do not want to disturb the memories of that time and place. I took away from that adventure with Margaret a greater willingness to try new things, and reconfirmed my budding commitment to "give back" to those who have helped me so much.

Now my home is on the side of Black Mountain in San Diego, and there are no forests like those of West Virginia. But there is a wonderful sunset to see each night as the sun sinks into the Pacific. It always reminds me of that special sunrise in West Virginia.

Judy Schmude, Ph.D., San Diego, CA.
Judy and Margaret were professional colleagues at Kenosha Memorial and maintained their friendship when Judy moved west – to Arizona and then to California. Their West Virginia trip was a special shared experience

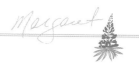

*S*eptember 7, 1999 6:15 a.m.

I thought about what I might add to what's been said. And I realized that what we knew best together was this 24 acres in Bayfield that we shared for such a short time. So I took a walk early this morning. And I want to tell you about it.

I wore the Spam hat that made you groan. Over a ponytail you never saw. Out the basement door and down the front yard. There's the bird-feeder that Rachael and Carl gave me. I've enjoyed watching the birds arrive and compete for the goodies. And despite the squirrel baffle, I get too many of them. A recent B&B guest, an avid bird-watcher, observed my frustration with the invaders and decided to send me a T-shirt with a front and profile view of a squirrel that says "wanted in 5 neighborhoods on 17 counts of larceny."

There's the fence we built to cover the utility equipment. The wild asparagus you saw in '96 is still growing. I walk along the gravel that Carl and Joel scattered Memorial Day weekend '96, just before we opened, and past the garden you and I cleared. The garden is full of underbrush, but the daffodils you planted appear each spring to announce the start of a new season.

I cross two planks over the little creek where the marsh marigolds bloom, and up the other side to where the trail you and Eva laid out begins to widen. I walk east about 50 feet where the wild...

...blackberry thickets tug at your clothes, then turn north where the apple trees appear. Droppings tell me the deer have been sampling the crop. I learned that these aren't volunteer trees as we thought, but that this used to be an orchard. The apples aren't much for looks, but if you eat around the spots, they're tasty.

On the right is where one solitary daffodil blooms each spring. Did you have something to do with that? On the left is the fern field that was such a surprise when we first discovered it in the spring of '95. It's turning from green to brown and will soon disappear for the winter.

Now east across the top of the trail, through grasses that were over my head just a few weeks ago, but are matted, perhaps starting to hunker down for the fall and winter ahead. Here's where the lupines begin. Their pods are dried and cracked, dropping seeds to assure an array of purple, lavender and white next spring. The birch tree that fell across the trail has been gradually whittled back over the last three years so that it no longer threatens to stab strollers – but I still keep a ribbon on it as a warning.

Turn right and start south, kicking apples off the trail. Over to the west about 100 feet is where we camped. The picnic table and fire pit are still there. So is the wood we cut. There's also a bench I made – crude, but comfortable – and dedicated to you June 14, 1998 to mark the second anniversary of our opening.

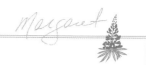

Just beyond that is the spot where you, Rachael, Eva, John, Karen and I joined to celebrate and pray that September morning in '96.

I stop at the artesian well. The water is still pouring out clear and cold, more than 4 gallons a minute. It was our cooking, drinking and washing water while we camped here after buying the land in '94 and during construction in '95.

Heading west again through the part that's almost impassible in mid-summer. Here's that big hunk of timber we dragged from the well in '96 to make a bridge across this little trickle of a stream. Here's the meadow where you, Kathy and your Dad and I sowed lupine seeds just about this time in '94. It's taken 5 years for them to take root and bloom. We had a dozen healthy clusters this June.
Some day this whole meadow may be full of lupines.

Remember the Charleston bench that was in front of our place in Madison? I painted it and moved it out here so people can sit and enjoy this meadow. It's very peaceful in spring, summer or fall.
Winter too, but then the bench disappears under the snow.

Now I'm at the driveway and heading up toward the house. Over on the right is where you planted your garden in '96 – you tended it as long as you could before it became too tiring. Stakes still mark its boundaries. The chives are still growing. The composter John Telford gave you is back there behind the trees, and I use it regularly. Remember when some animal – probably a bear – got into it just...

...after we moved in and I found it in four pieces in the morning?

Now around this last turn where the trees block your view for a moment . . . and then . . . here's the house.

It's everything we hoped it would be. You were right: the cedar needed to be stained silver-grey. It's weathered well. It wouldn't have looked right if we'd left it natural. But the deck will need to be re-done in 2000. Guests love the hammock.
(Two honeymooners fell asleep on it the other night).
I bought some 1950-style metal chairs to match the green trim and doors, and they look good.

Inside. The kitchen is wonderful. It's fine for one – would be better for two. But over time I've learned to put together a decent breakfast.

The great room is . . . a really great room. Remember that day when you stood right there in the center of the room and said , "What I'd like to do with this space is bring the outside inside."? Well, that's exactly the feeling you get. Sadly, you only saw summer and a bit of fall. But, whatever the season, we can look out the windows and truly feel part of nature. I've added a few new pieces in the room – some we might have had a spirited discussion about – but it's still basically what you and I put together.

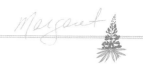

In fact, a recent guest wrote in the book:
"Our sense of Margaret's presence and continuing
'advisory role' here is strong and wonderful."

Your hats are on the rack, Brian's fireplace always draws
comments, and the wreath from your memorial service
will rest permanently on one of the beams.

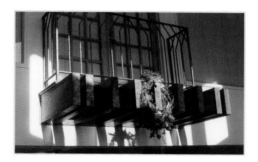

There's a framed poster from the 1998 Ragtime Night
at the Big Top. I asked that it be inscribed to both of us.
Remember, Ragtime Night was the only show we were able
to see in '96 – the only show you ever saw at the Tent.

I want you to know that guests invariably look at your picture
and say, "She was a beautiful woman."

And if guests don't write this in the book,
they always say it to me: "Her spirit is here."

– Al

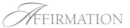

AFFIRMATION

One sunny February morning, more than a year after Margaret's
death, something told me to brew a pot of strong coffee, sit down
and look through a large box that had not been touched for some
15 months. The box contained get-well messages received
after Margaret had been diagnosed and sympathy cards
that arrived following her death.

Tucked in among the cards, I found a single sheet of her note
paper on which she had written – probably in September, 1996:

> *"Affirmation – When I go to sleep I instruct my
> body to continue its healing at an even higher
> intensity and I sense my body following these
> instructions. I tell this cancer these things:
> Thank you for teaching me to stop and listen;
> thank you for reminding me of what is truly
> important. You can go now. I know that I have
> things to do, gifts to give, projects to accom-
> plish, and I require a healthy working body for
> this. More and more I know that I will get well,
> not out of fear of dying. I will get well out of the
> joy of living."*

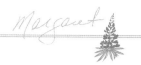

$\mathscr{A}$ND FINALLY . . .

It was October 18, 1998, the Sunday that marked the second
anniversary of Margaret's death. I wanted to celebrate the day
in a special way. I went to a local coffee house – one Margaret
never saw but would have loved – and ordered a cup to go.

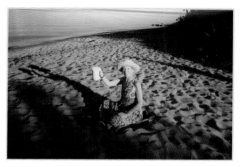

I drove to one of her favorite spots – a nearby beach on the
Lake Superior shore that is busy during the summer, but on this
gray, October afternoon was deserted. I drank coffee.
I remembered Margaret's last visit to this spot, pictured here.
And I scattered some of her ashes in the Big Lake she loved –
and enjoyed so briefly.

I drove back to our B&B and walked the land. As I turned
to head north up the highway toward Bayfield, something caught
my eye. There – blooming long beyond its May-June
growing season – was a single lupine. . .

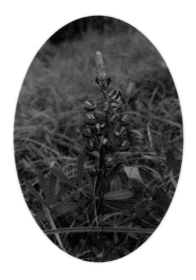

. . .And I knew that Margaret was there, too.

Al Chechik
October 18, 1999, Bayfield

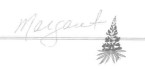

$\mathcal{U}$NDERSTANDING MARGARET

By now, I hope this book's words and pictures have helped
you form your own sense of Margaret.
You know what she looked like. You have read how and why she
affected the lives of others – in *their* words.

But, the closer I got to completing the book, the stronger
I felt that you, the reader, needed to have a sense of Margaret
as she moved toward the end of her journey in the late
summer/early fall of 1996.

You needed some understanding of what *she* was thinking.

So after much thought – and with the approval of its recipient –
I offer this letter. It's a clear, simple statement by a 49-year-old
woman who has much to live for, has inoperable cancer and has
been given very long odds for beating it. It is Margaret at her best
– articulate, realistic, hopeful and with an ironic touch of humor.

The letter was written to Janet Rigsbee Verstegen,
a longtime friend who lives in Little Chute, Wisconsin,
and grew up a block from Margaret.

SEPTEMBER 3, 1996

Dear Janet,

Thanks so much for your note and good thoughts.
I intended to respond much sooner, but my intentions
are greatly exceeding my energy these days.

I'm glad Kathy called and filled you in. There are a number
of people I wanted to get in touch with, but it is so difficult telling
each one. Especially when the conversations start out with the
other person saying something like "Great to hear from you.
What's new?"

It's been an incredible 5 weeks. I knew I was sick – loss
of weight, loss of appetite and then finally a lot of pain, but
I attributed it to the stress of moving, change in lifestyle, bad
eating and exercise routines during the months leading up to the
move. When Al moved up permanently in mid-June, I seemed
to get sicker faster, but again I thought it was just the mind telling
the body, "It's ok now. Help is here and you can take the time
to be sick." What I thought was that I had a virus or perhaps gall
bladder. Only in the darkest corner of my mind did the
word cancer even whisper.

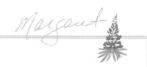

Now it's shouting. It's stomach cancer, quite advanced,
and we're working hard at beating it. My odds, by the way,
are 99.9% for a miracle cure. The other boring statistical medical
odds, I don't want to even think about.

Like most folks, the original confrontation put us into a state
of shock. I got an initial reading here (Ashland) and called my
doc in Madison. Got set up with an oncologist in Madison and
came down the next day (a Friday). He told me to go back
to Bayfield and clear the decks for at least two weeks to return
to Madison and get a definitive diagnosis, then discuss alternatives
and begin treatment. At that time, and through the first couple
days of tests, we were all hopeful it was lymphoma. Unfortunately,
that turned out to not be the case, but rather stomach cancer.

The how and why questions call out to be answered, but there are
no simple answers. Why me, why now, why this kind of cancer.
For me, the focus is more on: what next? I have it, it's big, bad
and ugly, and I want to overcome it. Our plan is to pursue the
usual medical treatment route in hopes of a brief remission. If we
can get that, we'll have time to put alternative healing searches
into place. My oncologist is an extraordinary guy (would I accept
anything but extraordinary?) who is willing to work with massage,
nutrition, mental/spiritual, anything that helps me. He's been very
forthright about how little standard medical practice can offer me

at this time, yet how he knows of and acknowledges
non-medical "cures" of people living active lives after medical
science gave up and sent them home to die.

I'm not ready to die yet. Life is so good, there is so much
yet to be experienced and shared in with others I care about,
that I believe this journey is not yet ended.

So, yes, The Artesian House is open and accepting reservations.
And, of course, I would love to have you and any others from
the old gang come share this special place. These days, Al is doing
most of the work. My energy is strongly depleted by the combo
of chemo and cancer, so he has had to pick up a big share of the
cooking and cleaning. I still spend time with the guests,
but it is limited. Right now, we are trying to keep those good
moments for ourselves and family and friends who visit.

We've had great emergency backup from our families.
Al's youngest son, Joel, with wife Sara and baby Lucy, came up
and ran the place for four days when we first went to Madison.
Al's sister and brother-in-law were in California at the time on
vacation, so they cut it short to spend the last week running the
Artesian House and then helping us get settled back in. Worked
out great as Al's sister is an oncology nurse and bringing home
a cancer patient for the first time after being surrounded
by the security of hospital staff is a little like the first days home

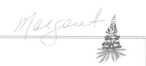

with a baby! We go down to Madison on Tuesday for the next
round of chemo, and we'll just close up for the week days
(the mid-week season goes down sharply after Labor Day)
and Al's other son and lady are coming up from St. Louis next
Friday to hold down the fort until we get back Sunday.
Last weekend Rachael came up to help Al as cleaning staff.
We're currently looking for someone locally to come
in for a few hours each Saturday and Sunday to give
Al cleaning backup. So things fall into place as they need to.

This is turning into a much longer "note" than I started
out to write. But you know it has always been helpful for me
to write/talk things out, and I thank you for reading/listening.
And even if you're not, one of the advantages of writing over the
telephone call is I can THINK you're following along, even
if you're not. Also, rambling, as I am doing now, is much
cheaper by letter than by phone.

In many ways, Janet, this has been among the most wonderful
times of my life. My marriage has always been strong; now
I can't begin to articulate the depth of our feelings for each other.
Without Al in my life, I don't know how I would face this
challenge. With him, every moment has significance. With
Rachael, it has been so difficult to watch her struggle with the
situation. We are deeply bound, as only children can be, and even

more so since I single-parented her for so many years.
Our love is such a special gift, but with it comes the higher price
of pain and loss – for both of us. I can't even begin to
contemplate not being part of her future, not watching her grow
each day into a more beautiful person. Family and friends have
responded beyond any reasonable expectations in terms of love
and support. Like yourself, so many have reached out to me.
And from you all, I derive strength and courage…
and determination. If this many really terrific people
really do think I'm terrific too, then by golly, I intend
to stick around to enjoy.

Each day, I do a visualization that involves all who love and
care for me, present or passed beyond, gathering around
me in a special healing place to lend their energy and strength
to my healing efforts. Each day, Janet, I hope you'll place yourself
in that circle and lend me some of your strength.

Pass on to Lynn (Diesel) my thanks for her prayers. And to
any others who ask what they might do, to pray in their own way
to their own he/she/it/them/us/other that I may stay the course
with strength, courage, determination and a sense of humor, and
that I may be healed. (As you can see, I am still having trouble
with that god thing. I think I see why the Jews went to yahweh
rather than naming their deity.)

Margaret

Thanks Janet, for being Janet.
Over all the years, we have always been able to maintain that common bond that remains strong. And I have always known that if I ever needed a friend, I could call on you. And I do, and I did and, of course, you responded.

Margaret

P.S. Did you know a wig for a cancer patient is now called a "cranial prosthesis." Oh the wonders of reimbursement. A wig is not reimbursable, but a cranial prosthesis can be.